Aids to Fluid and Electrolyt

Aids to Fluid and Electrolyte Balance

Norman Muirhead

MD, MRCP, FRCP(C)

Assistant Professor of Medicine/Nephrology, University of Western Ontario, London, Ontario, Canada

Graeme R. D. Catto

MD, FRCP, FRCPGlasg

Reader in Medicine, University of Aberdeen; Honorary Consultant Physician/Nephrologist, Grampian Health Board, Aberdeen, UK

CHURCHILL LIVINGSTONE
EDINBURGH LONDON MELBOURNE AND NEW YORK 1986

CHURCHILL LIVINGSTONE
Medical Division of Longman Group UK Limited

Distributed in the United States of America by
Churchill Livingstone Inc., 1560 Broadway, New
York, N.Y. 10036, and by associated companies,
branches and representatives throughout the
world.

First published 1986

ISBN 0 443 03609 8

British Library Cataloguing in Publication Data
Muirhead, Norman
  Aids to fluid and electrolyte balance.
  1. Water-electrolyte imbalances
  I. Title   II. Catto, Graeme R. D.
  616.3′9   RC630

Library of Congress Cataloging in Publication Data
Muirhead, Norman.
  Aids to fluid and electrolyte balance.
  Includes index.
  Water-electrolyte imbalances — Outlines,
syllabi, etc. 2. Water-electrolyte balance
(Physiology) — Outlines, syllabi, etc. I. Catto,
Graeme R. D. II. Title. [DNLM: 1. Water-
Electrolyte Balance. QU 105 M953a]
  RC630.M85 1986 616.3′986-12970

Produced by Longman Singapore Publishers (Pte) Ltd.
Printed in Singapore

Preface

This is a concise textbook for all with an interest in the clinical management of fluid and electrolyte balance. It is designed principally to meet the needs of young clinicians, both physicians and surgeons, preparing for postgraduate qualifications but should also prove useful for interested medical students during their clinical training.

Physiological concepts are outlined and contrasted with pathophysiological conditions found in clinical practice. In this way the text provides a bridge between the principles of physiology and the practical management of patients with a wide variety of conditions. The chapters are succinct and well tabulated with much of the information contained in tables and figures. A series of illustrative clinical problems, together with appropriate answers, is included at the end of the book.

London, Ontario and Aberdeen, 1986   N. M.
                                                                                          G. R. D. C.

Contents

Contents

Introduction

BODY FLUIDS

In a healthy individual water comprises approximately 60% of total body weight and is generally considered to be divided into two main compartments—intracellular and extracellular fluid. The extracellular fluid compartment may in turn be subdivided into interstitial and intravascular fluids. Approximately two-thirds of total body water is intracellular and the remainder is extracellular; two-thirds of the extracellular fluid is interstitial and the remainder intravascular. Thus (Fig. 1) in a 70 kg normal adult with approximately 42 litres of total body water, 28 litres are intracellular and 14 litres extracellular; of the extracellular fluid, 4 litres are intravascular (plasma volume) and the remainder extravascular and interstitial.

Water has small, highly diffusible molecules which are polar, so that they cohere with one another making the substance liquid rather than gas, as well as having other vital thermal

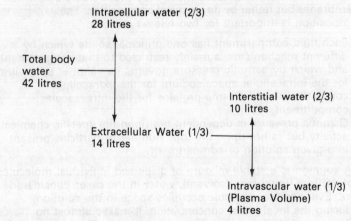

Fig. 1 Distribution of body water in a 70 kg man.

properties. Water is a first-class solvent, for its molecules associate with (i.e. 'hydrate') proteins, sugars and many other solutes especially ions, greatly modifying their properties and separating and dispersing (dissolving) them. Water itself ionises very slightly, the $[H^+]$ of neutral water being 10^{-7} g.ion/l (pH 7). Water is abundant in the body; not only is it about 60% by weight—it accounts for something over 90% of the molecules of the body.

Movement of molecules is by bulk flow and by diffusion, the direction of which is determined by any spatial difference of concentration or force which can be summed up as a *gradient*. A gradient can be thought of as a notional 'slope' which things have to go 'down' at a rate depending on its 'steepness'.

Bulk flow is the concerted movement of the solution mass in the direction of a hydrostatic pressure gradient at a rate depending also on the mechanical resistance to flow. *Diffusion* is the result of random individual molecular movements whose effect is to disperse a local accumulation of any molecular species if it is free to move. This means substances tend to move down any available concentration gradients. Diffusion on its own is only important in liquids over rather short distances though it is speedy in gases, but is fundamental to an understanding of osmosis. *Osmosis* can be understood as the diffusional movement of *solvent* down its own concentration gradient, a gradient created by inequality of *solute* distribution (see below).

Osmotic pressure
The volume of each compartment is determined not simply by the quantity of water present which may move freely across cell membranes but rather by its chemical composition. The composition is important for two related reasons:

1. Each fluid compartment has one principal solute which by different mechanisms is mainly restricted to that compartment and which by osmotic pressure governs its volume: potassium for the intracellular space sodium for the extracellular compartment and plasma proteins for the intravascular compartment.
2. Osmotic pressure is dependent not upon the specific chemical activity but rather upon the total number of particles present in a given solution or compartment.

A solution is a stable mixture of dispersed individual molecules (solute) in a liquid bulk (solvent), water in the cases considered here. Every solute molecule occupies space in the solution, reducing the local water concentration. It makes almost no difference what particular solute molecule it is. The water molecules share the general property of all molecules that they undergo net movement by diffusion down their gradient of concentration. They will therefore tend to diffuse from a region of low total solute concentration (that is, high solvent concentration) to one of higher total solute concentration (lower solvent concentration). The extent of this tendency for solvent to move can be measured in an apparatus which prevents solute movement (a semi-permeable membrane) by means of the hydrostatic pressure required to produce an equal and opposite bulk flow to the diffusional solvent flow. This equivalent pressure is called the osmotic pressure of the solution, and is approximately proportional to the sum of the concentrations of all the solute particles present.

In practice, the measurement of osmotic activity is made more easily by the effect of total solute concentration in depressing the freezing point of the solution. The units of osmotic activity (corresponding to the sum of the molar quantities of all the solutes if they could be known) are called osmoles (osm). Ionic compounds exert osmotic activity proportional to the number of particles into which they dissociate. For instance a 100 mM solution of a non-ionic compound (e.g. glucose) would exert about the same osmotic pressure as a 50 mM solution of a compound fully dissociating into two ions per mole (e.g. NaCl) or 33 mM of a compound yielding three (e.g. $CaCl_2$). Though it is possible to express osmotic activity per litre of solution, osmolarity, there are advantages, notably in temperature independence of the unit, in using osmoles per kg of water, osmolality. An osmolality of 1 osm/kg exerts an osmotic pressure of 22.4 atmospheres and lowers the freezing point by 1.86°C. The practical osmotic pressure units for body fluids are mosm/kg. Apart from the renal medulla (see below), the normal osmolality of cells and body fluids is just under 300 mosm/kg.

The volumes of body compartments are determined by the solute contents of the compartments, since with certain important exceptions to be mentioned, the boundaries are permeable to water but much less permeable to particular solutes. Water therefore flows across the boundaries until the balance of osmotic and hydrostatic forces falls to zero.

BODY FLUID COMPARTMENTS

Intravascular compartment (plasma)

The proteins normally present in plasma in a concentration of 70–80 g/l (7–8 g/100 ml) do not form a single homogeneous group. Albumin with a concentration of 40–50 g/l (4–5 g/100 ml) forms the largest single component whereas the remainder, the globulins, are both more diverse and larger. Because of its plasma concentration and low molecular weight (68 000 d) albumin produces almost 80% of the oncotic pressure (colloid osmotic pressure) of the plasma. However even at best this pressure amounts only to 0.7 m osmol/kg water.

$$\frac{\text{Plasma concentration (g/l)}}{\text{molecular weight}} = \frac{50}{68\,000} = 0.7 \text{ mmol (or mosm/l)}$$

The normal serum osmolality of 290 mosm is produced mainly by such small solutes (crystalloids) as sodium chloride, glucose and urea which can cross freely from the intravascular to the interstitial compartment as the capillary basement membrane is semi-permeable. The plasma proteins, because of their large molecular weight and size, are unable to leave the intravascular (plasma) space and thus cause the only effective osmotic pressure difference between plasma and the interstitial extracellular fluid—the colloid osmotic pressure. As first proposed by Starling, this small pressure difference opposes the hydrostatic pressure produced in the capillary network by the systemic blood pressure and tends to draw fluid back into the intravascular compartment and thus maintain both the plasma volume and a continuous circulation of tissue fluid. At the arterial end of the capillary, the hydrostatic pressure is greater than the plasma oncotic pressure and thus favours the formation of the protein-free interstitial fluid. The opposite pressure effect occurs at the venous end of the capillary where colloid osmotic pressure overcomes the reduced hydrostatic pressure and tissue fluid is drawn back into the intravascular space. In this way the plasma protein concentration permits the heart to pump only one-third of the extracellular fluid as the circulating plasma volume and still obtain a continuous circulation of the entire interstitial fluid which bathes the cells of the body. The small quantities of plasma protein and fluid which leak from the capillaries are returned to the systemic circulation by the lymphatic system.

THE INTRACELLULAR AND EXTRACELLULAR FLUIDS

Mainly because of the difficulties involved in obtaining samples of the fluid relatively little is known about the control of the intracellular fluid volume in health or disease. However, as two-thirds of the total body water is intracellular and as body weight varies by only 1–2% daily, a precise form of control must exist. Moreover, as the cell membranes are freely permeable to water and large macromolecules which exert an osmotic gradient are contained within the cells, some mechanism must be present to prevent unrestricted entry of water with subsequent swelling of the cells, which, unlike plant cells, are not surrounded by a tough membrane.

To prevent the cell continuing to swell until either it ruptures or its contents are considerably diluted, it must be able to export water. Every animal cell in which the search has been made has been found to possess at least one important mechanism, namely a membrane-bound Na^+/K^+ exchanger. This works because the sodium ion happens to bind more water than the potassium ion. This alone would dictate that exporting sodium ion in exchange for potassium ion would also export water. The important point, however, is that though sodium has the smaller atom, the hydrated sodium ion is larger than the hydrated potassium ion, so sodium leaks into cells less readily than potassium leaks out. The movement of a hydrated sodium ion is not only more restricted than that of potassium, but when it does move in a restricted pore, it entrains the movement of a great deal more water than does the smaller ion.

The consequence of the presence of the Na^+/K^+ exchanger is that Na^+ accumulates in the extracellular space and K^+ inside cells to the extent of about 140 mM, while the concentrations of Na^+ inside and K^+ outside are usually under 10 mM. The rate of entry of Na^+ is limited by a low membrane permeability to Na^+, but the rate of escape of K^+ is limited not by the membrane permeability to K^+ but the inability of the predominantly anionic macromolecules to escape. Outward leak of the permeant K^+ therefore tends to separate the cell's charges to a minute degree, causing the outside of the cell to become positively charged almost enough to prevent further K^+ exit. This means that Na^+ extrusion take place not only against a substantial chemical concentration gradient, but also against the electrical gradient. The Na^+/K^+ exchanger therefore has to use substantial amounts of energy in the form of ATP. The mechanism is thus often referred to as an Na^+/K^+-ATPase. This generates one of the major energy demands of the cell, and one that is sensitive to both hypoxia and H^+ changes.

Normal sodium and water homeostasis

WATER HOMEOSTASIS

Control of water intake

This depends on the integrity of the central thirst mechanism. Serious disorders of water homeostasis are therefore unusual in the conscious adult with free access to water. Thirst is mediated by anterior hypothalamic receptors and is stimulated by increased serum osmolality (usually due to hypernatraemia or more rarely hyperglycaemia). Reduction in serum osmolality (usually due to hyponatraemia) suppresses thirst.

Control of water output

Renal water excretion depends on a number of factors including the normal operation of renal mechanisms involved in urinary dilution and concentration, the sodium status of the individual and anti-diuretic hormone (ADH) status.

1. *Urinary dilution and concentration* depends on the interplay between the renal medullary countercurrent multiplier system and ADH. The normal operation of the countercurrent multiplier system is illustrated in Figure 2. The maximum medullary osmotic gradient that can be achieved by the human kidney is around 900 mosm/kg water giving a final urinary concentration of 1200 mosm/kg water (900 mosm/kg water + plasma ultrafiltrate osmolality of 300 mosm/kg water). Medullary hypertonicity is achieved largely by active transport of chloride (with passive sodium transport to maintain electrical neutrality) out of the ascending loop of Henle. This hypertonicity is maintained by countercurrent exchange in the vasa recta (Fig. 3) where low rates of blood flow and passive movement of sodium, chloride and urea into the hypertonic interstitium prevent solute washout.

   Tubular fluid leaving the loop of Henle is hypotonic with respect to plasma. In the absence of ADH the medullary collecting ducts remain impermeable to water and a dilute urine is excreted. In the presence of ADH the medullary collecting ducts are permeable to water and water

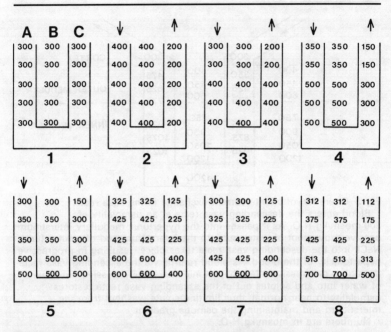

Fig. 2 Operation of the countercurrent multiplier system.
A = descending loop of Henle; B = interstitium; C = ascending loop of
Henle. 1. The loop of Henle is filled with isosmotic fluid. 2. NaCl is
actively reabsorbed from the ascending loop of Henle, which is
impermeable to water, to produce a difference of 200 mosm/kg H_2O at
each level. The descending loop of Henle is freely permeable to water
and equilibrates with the medullary interstitium. 3. As more isosmotic
fluid is added, hyposmolar fluid exits into the distal tubule. 4. Further
reabsorption of NaCl reestablishes the 200 mosm/kg H_2O differential 5–8.
Further addition of isosmotic fluid and reabsorption of NaCl in the
ascending limb leads to progressive increase in medullary interstitial
hypertonicity.

reabsorption will occur due to the hypertonicity of the
medullary interstitium. Maximum water conservation thereby
occurs and a concentrated urine is excreted.
2. *Sodium status.* Sodium intake plays an important role in
determining water excretion. Excess dietary sodium is filtered
at the glomerulus (see p. 12) and delivered to the proximal
tubule. Proximal sodium reabsorption is depressed (40% vs.
67%) in salt-loading states due to poorly understood factors
(e.g. natriuretic hormone) and increased amounts of sodium
and water are delivered distally. Urine flow rate is thereby
increased and, since distal sodium reabsorption is also
impaired, a natriuresis and water diuresis will occur.

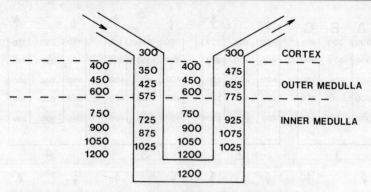

Fig. 3 Operation of countercurrent exchange in the vasa recta.
Blood enters the descending vasa recta at an osmolality of
300 mosm/kg H_2O. As it passes into the hypertonic medullary interstitium
passive movement of water out into the interstitium and of solutes (urea,
NaCl) into the descending vasa recta takes place, resulting in progressive
hypertonicity of the blood. As blood returns via the ascending vasa recta
through a progressively less hypertonic interstitium, passive movement
of water into and solutes out of the ascending vasa recta restores
osmolality to near normal, thus limiting solute washout from the
interstitium and maintaining the osmotic gradient.
Numbers are in mosm/kg H_2O.

3. *ADH* is a cyclic octapeptide that is synthesised in the
   supraoptic nucleus of the hypothalamus and conveyed by an
   axonal delivery system to the posterior pituitary where it is
   stored and released in response to a number of stimuli. The
   physiological control of ADH release and suppression is
   summarised in Table 1. Under normal circumstances serum
   osmolality is maintained within narrow limits. However, when
   plasma volume falls by 10% or more, non-osmotic (mainly
   volume and baroreceptor) stimuli predominate and maintain
   plasma volume at the expense of any change in serum
   osmolality.

Osmolar and free water clearance
Total water output is made up of two theoretical quantities,
osmolar clearance (C_{osm} = the amount of water required to
excrete solutes at the concentration of solute in plasma) and free
water clearance (^cH_2O = the amount of water that must be
added to hypertonic urine or subtracted from hypotonic urine to
render the urine isotonic). Thus hypertonic urine gives a negative
free water clearance which measures water conservation.

$$C_{osm} = U_{osm} \times \text{urine flow } (V)/P_{osm;} \; ; \; V = C_{osm} + {}^cH_2O$$

The average solute load on a normal Western diet is around
600 mosm/24 hours. Since maximum urinary concentration is

Table 1 Physiological control of ADH secretion

ADH secretion ↑	ADH secretion ↓

Increased plasma osmolality
  hypernatraemia
  hyperglycaemia
  mannitol
	Decreased plasma osmolality
	  hyponatremia

Volume contraction
  left atrial/venous capacitance
receptors
	Volume expansion
	  left atrial/venous capacitance
	receptors

Hypotension
  aortic baroreceptors
  left atrial receptors
	Hypertension
	  aortic baroreceptors

Autonomic stimuli due to
  pain/stress
  hypoxia
  liver disease	

1200 mosm/kg water a minimum urine volume of 500 ml/24 hours is required to excrete a normal solute load.

$$C_{osm} = \frac{UV}{P} = \frac{1200 \text{ mosm/kg H}_2\text{O} . 500 \text{ ml/24 hours}}{300 \text{ mosm/kg/H}_2\text{O}}$$

$$= 2000 \text{ ml/24 hours}$$

$V = C_{osm} + {}^cH_2O$ ${}^cH_2O$ is negative in this case (i.e. water has been reabsorbed). A negative ${}^cH_2O$ is given the term T^cH_2O.

$$T^cH_2O = C_{osm} - V$$
$$= 2000 - 500 \text{ ml/24 hours}$$
$$= 1500 \text{ ml/24 hours}$$

∴ only 1500 ml of solute free water was added to the body during maximal antidiuresis.

In a situation of maximum urinary dilution U_{osm} may be 60 mosm/kg water and urine volume 10 l/24 hours. In this situation:

$$C_{osm} = \frac{60 \text{ mosm/kg H}_2\text{O} . 10000 \text{ ml/24 hours}}{300 \text{ mosm/kg H}_2\text{O}}$$

$$= 2000 \text{ ml/day}$$

$$V = C_{osm} + {}^cH_2O$$

$$\therefore {}^cH_2O = 10000 - 2000 \text{ ml}$$
$$= 8 \text{ l}$$

i.e. 8 l of free water has been added to the urine.

The concept of free water clearance is of little clinical significance but does help in understanding primary disorders of water homeostasis. The examples show the much greater power of the kidney to compensate for excessive rather than deficient water intake. It is virtually impossible therefore for major disturbances in plasma sodium or water to be induced purely by voluntary means unless the usual homeostatic mechanism has been subverted, for example by inappropriate ADH secretion (see below), by renal or circulatory failure, or by gross over-infusion of dextrose.

SODIUM HOMEOSTASIS

Total body sodium
Normal total body sodium is around 5000 mmol of which about 60% is freely exchangeable. Much of the non-exchangeable sodium is in bone. Most of total body sodium is extracellular (3500–4000 mmol) and may be measured directly by a whole body counting technique. Exchangeable sodium can be measured by isotope dilution techniques. Such measurements are rarely practical in the clinical setting and are used principally in research.

A rough estimation of total body sodium in clinical practice is possible by physical examination. In general, oedema states are associated with an increased total body sodium irrespective of the serum sodium which is, in fact, frequently low in these circumstances (see below). Similarly, low total body sodium is usually accompanied by evidence of ECF volume depletion viz. postural hypotension and dehydration (see below) irrespective of serum sodium, which is often high.

Normal sodium intake and output
The average sodium content of the normal Western diet is around 155 mmol/24 hours. Of this around 2.5 mmol are excreted in sweat and in faeces, the remaining 150 mmol being excreted via the kidneys. In the absence of significant extrarenal losses (e.g. diarrhoea, sweating) urinary sodium in general reflects dietary sodium intake.

Renal sodium handling (Fig. 4)
1. *Glomerular filtration.* Sodium is freely filtered at the glomerulus and is delivered to the proximal tubule in proportion to its plasma concentration.
2. *Proximal tubule.* Around two-thirds of filtered sodium is reabsorbed isotonically with chloride in the proximal tubule. This involves active sodium transport. Reduction of GFR or increased proximal sodium reabsorption may reduce distal

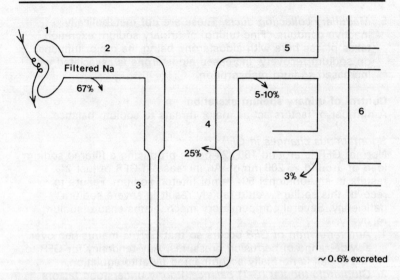

Fig. 4 Renal tubular Na reabsorption. Normally ~ 25 000 mmol Na/24 hours filtered while urinary Na is 150 mmol/24 hours or less. 1. Glomerulus; 2. Proximal tubule; 3. Thin descending limb loop of Henle; 4. Thick ascending limb loop of Henle; 5. Distal tubule; 6. Collecting duct.

sodium and water delivery. This can interfere with normal urinary dilution and concentration, reducing the maximum medullary concentration gradient that can be achieved by limiting the hypotonicity of the fluid delivered to the distal tubule (see p. 6).

3. *Loop of Henle*. Chloride is actively reabsorbed in the thick ascending limb of the loop of Henle, sodium moving passively to maintain electrical neutrality. In this way around 25% of filtered sodium is reabsorbed in the loop of Henle. Since this region of the nephron is impermeable to water this process results in progressive hypotonicity of the tubular fluid. This is the major method of dilute urine production since beyond this point additional net sodium reabsorption is possible only in the absence of ADH. Chloride and sodium reabsorption from the ascending limb is also important in permitting urinary concentration as it contributes to maintaining the integrity of the medullary concentration gradient (see Fig. 2).

4. *Distal tubule*. In normal circumstances around 5–10% of filtered sodium (1260–2520 mmol) reaches distal sites of reabsorption. The precise mechanism of sodium reabsorption at this site is unknown though some sodium is exchanged for potassium or hydrogen ion under the influence of aldosterone (see below).

5. *Medullary collecting ducts.* These are not metabolically
   inactive conduits. 'Fine-tuning' of urinary sodium excretion
   takes places here with aldosterone being the major influence
   on sodium recovery. Increased aldosterone is associated with
   increased sodium reabsorption.

Control of urinary sodium excretion
A number of factors act as major threats to sodium balance.

Spontaneous changes in GFR
Normal GFR is around 180 l/24 hours producing a filtered sodium
load of around 25 200 mmol. An increase in GFR of just 2%
results in an additional 504 mmol filtered sodium. Failure to
recover this sodium would rapidly result in severe sodium
deficiency. Several compensatory mechanisms ensure sodium
recovery.
1. *Autoregulation of GFR* occurs so that GFR is maintained over
   a wide range of perfusion pressures. Any tendency for GFR to
   rise or fall is normally accompanied by autoregulation.
2. *Glomerulo-tubular (G-T) balance.* Poorly understood factors
   (perhaps including concentration of solute delivered to the
   macula densa) feed back to maintain fractional proximal
   tubular sodium reabsorption at the normal two-thirds thus
   recovering additional filtered sodium. (Normal = 25 200 mmol;
   2% increase = 25 704 mmol; normal reabsorption = 25 200 ×
   0.67 = 16 884 mmol; G-T balance increases reabsorption to
   25 704 × 0.67 = 17 222 mmol, i.e. 17 222 − 16 884 =
   338 mmol additional sodium reabsorbed.)
   In the example given above G-T balance leaves 504 − 338 =
166 mmol additional sodium to be recovered in the loop of Henle
or at distal sites. This is well within the reabsorptive capacity of
distal sites.
   Both autoregulation of GFR and G-T balance operate under
physiological circumstances to ensure that spontaneous
variations in GFR do not inevitably lead to catastrophic changes
in urinary sodium excretion.

Variation in sodium intake
In general urinary sodium reflects dietary sodium intake as,
under normal circumstances, the kidneys are the major route of
sodium excretion. Variations in sodium intake are accompanied
by appropriate changes in urinary sodium excretion mediated by
one or more of the following:
1. *Increased GFR.* Sodium loading leads to a natriuresis that is
   mediated, at least in part, by an increased GFR. Unlike
   spontaneous change in GFR, changes in GFR induced by
   sodium loading or depletion are not accompanied by
   significant autoregulation or G-T balance.

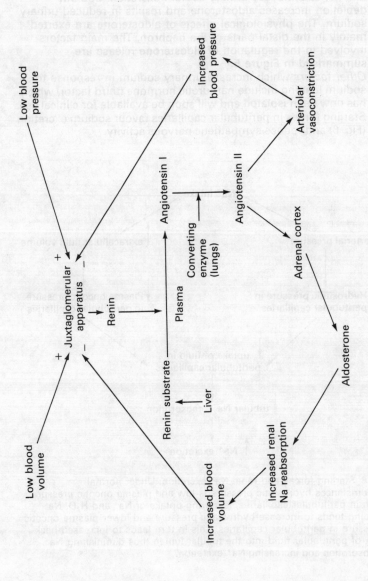

Fig. 5 Physiological control of renin-angiotension-aldosterone system

2. *Aldosterone.* Sodium loading suppresses aldosterone secretion and hence enhances urinary sodium excretion. Sodium depletion increases aldosterone and results in reduced urinary sodium. The physiological effects of aldosterone are exerted mainly in the distal parts of the nephron. The main factors involved in the regulation of aldosterone release are summarised in Figure 5.
3. *Other factors* which increase urinary sodium in response to sodium loading include natriuretic hormone (third factor) which has now been isolated and will soon be available for clinical use. Starling forces in peritubular capillaries favour sodium excretion (Fig. 6) and reduce sympathetic nervous activity.

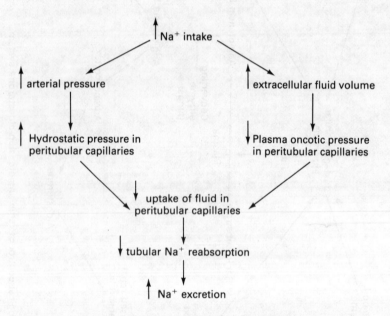

Fig.6 Starling forces and renal Na^+ excretion. Under normal circumstances hydrostatic pressure is low and plasma oncotic pressure high in peritubular capillaries, favouring uptake of Na^+ and H_2O. Na^+ loading tends to increase hydrostatic pressure and lower plasma oncotic pressure in peritubular capillaries. This in turn leads to increased back-leak of peritubular fluid into the tubular lumen thus diminishing Na^+ reabsorption and increasing Na^+ excretion.

Disorders of sodium and water homeostasis

Disorders of sodium and water homeostasis are complexly intertwined and therefore best discussed together as causing either hyponatraemia or hypernatraemia.

HYPONATRAEMIA

Hyponatraemia may present in a wide range of clinical settings and its detection should lead to a structured approach to diagnosis and therapy. The major causes of hyponatraemia are:
1. Severe CCF
2. Liver failure
3. Nephrotic syndrome
4. Acute/chronic renal failure
5. Endocrine
   a. Addison's disease—glucocorticoid deficiency
   b. hypopituitarism
   c. hypothyroidism
   d. inappropriate ADH (SIADH)
6. Extrarenal losses
   a. vomiting
   b. diarrhoea
   c. 'third space'—e.g. burns
   d. pancreatitis
7. Renal losses
   a. diuretics
   b. salt-losing nephritis; bicarbonaturia—e.g. RTA, metabolic alkalosis
   c. ketonuria—e.g. diabetes, alcohol, starvation
   d. osmotic diuresis e.g. glucose; urea; mannitol
8. Pseudohyponatraemia
   a. hyperlipidaemia
   b. myeloma
   c. Waldenstrom's macroglobulinaemia
   d. sampling from IV infusion arm
9. Osmolar shift—hyperglycaemia

Symptoms and signs of hyponatraemia
Symptoms
1. Lethargy
2. Confusion
3. Muscle cramps
4. Anorexia
5. Nausea
6. Agitation

Signs
1. Abnormal sensorium
2. Depressed reflexes
3. Cheyne-Strokes respiration
4. Hypothermia
5. Extensor plantar reflexes
6. Pseudobulbar palsy
7. Seizures
8. Coma and death

The major symptoms and signs of hyponatraemia are non-specific so that a high index of clinical suspicion is necessary in patients with disease states known to produce electrolyte disturbances. In general gastrointestinal symptoms predominate in mild and early hyponatraemia with CNS signs and symptoms occurring in severe and late hyponatraemia. Acute hyponatraemia causes more symptoms because of the accompanying acute increase in cerebral water content, while chronic hyponatraemia may produce little in the way of clinical features, even if the serum sodium is around 110 mmol/l. Hyponatraemia is also less well tolerated in the elderly.

Diagnosis of hyponatraemia
The first step is to rule out pseudohyponatraemia or hyponatraemia due to osmolar shift (usually due to hyperglycaemia). Pseudohyponatraemia occurs in lipid or protein disorders. Sodium is measured in whole plasma though it is present only in plasma water. If lipids or protein occupy an increased plasma volume; e.g. in hyperlipidaemia or myeloma; sodium will be falsely low if measured in whole plasma. This problem can be eliminated by measuring sodium in plasma water after ultracentrifugation to remove excess plasma solids. If ultracentrifugation is not available it is more practical to measure plasma osmolality. Plasma osmolality is low in true hyponatraemia and normal in psuedohyponatraemia.

Hyponatraemia during hyperglycaemia occurs as a result of the increased number of osmotically active glucose molecules (which do not penetrate well into cells in the absence of insulin) in the

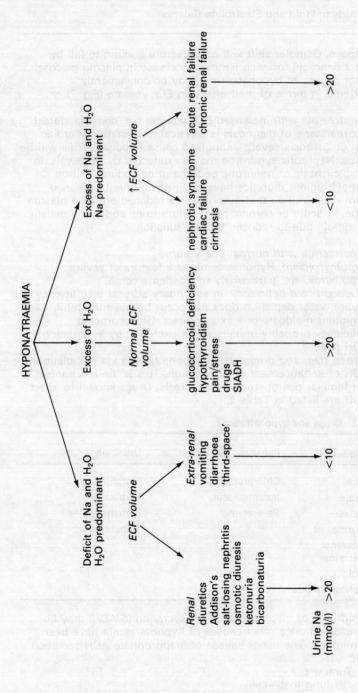

Fig. 7 Diagnosis of hyponatraemia based on assessment of ECF volume status and urinary sodium.

ECF space. Osmolar shift will cause serum sodium to fall by about 1.6 mmol/l for each 6 mmol/l increase in plasma glucose.

Other causes of hyponatraemia may be conveniently considered in terms of their effect on ECF volume (Fig. 7).

Hyponatraemia with increased ECF volume (i.e. oedema states)
The cornerstone of diagnosis is physical examination. Cardiac failure or cirrhosis severe enough to cause hyponatraemia will be obvious. Nephrotic syndrome may be detected by urinalysis. In cardiac, cirrhotic or nephrotic oedema urine sodium will be < 10 mmol/l, unless diuretics have been given, due to the avid sodium reabsorption that accompanies reduced effective plasma volume. In acute or chronic renal failure urine sodium is usually > 20 mmol/l due to reduced tubular function.

Hyponatraemia with normal ECF volume
1. *Hypothyroidism.* Hyponatraemia is a feature of severe hypothyroidism, particularly myxoedema coma.
2. *Glucocorticoid deficiency.* In secondary adrenal insufficiency severe water depletion does not occur because the renin-angiotensin-aldosterone axis is intact. Glucocorticoid deficiency probably impairs water excretion by enchancing ADH release.
3. *Stress, pain and drugs* cause hyponatraemia via stimulation of ADH or enhancement of ADH action. This is the mechanism of the familiar postoperative antidiuresis. Drugs known to affect ADH are listed in Table 2.

Table 2 Drugs and hyponatraemia

Stimulate ADH	Enhance ADH action	Unknown
Nicotine	Chlorpropamide	Morphine
Clofibrate	Indomethacin	Barbiturates
Vincristine	Paracetamol	Carbamazepine
Vinblastine		Tolbutamide
Isoproterenol (isoprenaline)		
Alcohol		
Cyclophosphamide		

4. *Syndrome of inappropriate ADH secretion (SIADH)* may be considered once other causes of hyponatraemia have been eliminated. The major causes of inappropriate ADH secretion are:
   a. Tumours
      (i) lung (oat—cell)

      (ii) duodenum
     (iii) pancreas
     (iv) lymphoma
      (v) thymoma
  b. Pulmonary
       (i) viral/bacterial pneumonia
      (ii) lung abscess
     (iii) empyema
     (iv) TB
      (v) aspergillosis
  c. CNS
       (i) meningitis—viral, bacterial or TB
      (ii) encephalitis—viral, bacterial
     (iii) acute psychosis
     (iv) cerebral haemorrhage/thrombosis/embolism
      (v) tumours—primary or secondary
     (vi) brain abscess
    (vii) CNS trauma—open/closed
   (viii) subdural/subarachnoid haemorrhage
     (ix) Guillain—Barre syndrome
      (x) acute intermittent porphyria
     (xi) systemic lupus

Hyponatraemia and decreased ECF volume
Urine sodium provides the major diagnostic clue: urine sodium
>20 mmol/l suggests renal sodium and water losses while urine
sodium < 10 mmol/l suggests extra-renal sodium and water
losses.

1. *Gastrointestinal and 'third space' losses.* The diagnosis is
   usually readily obvious from the clinical history. Diagnostic
   problems may occur in surreptitious vomiting or laxative
   abuse. In these cases there is usually a severe metabolic
   alkalosis and the urine is free of chloride. Urinary sodium is
   invariably low unless there is continued vomiting when the
   bicarbonaturia that accompanies the metabolic alkalosis will
   cause some increase in urinary sodium (see below).
   'Third space' (i.e. non-renal, non GI) losses are usually
   obvious from the clinical situation, e.g. severe burn,
   pancreatitis, extensive soft tissue injury.
2. *Renal losses* of sodium occur in a variety of circumstances.
   a. *Diuretics.* Overdiuresis is a common cause of
      hyponatraemia, usually accompanied by hypokalaemic
      metabolic alkalosis. Abuse of diuretics for weight loss is
      now common. Such patients may be distinguished from
      those with surreptitious vomiting or laxative abuse by
      the urine chloride which is > 20 mmol/l during diuretic
      therapy.

b. *Salt-losing nephritis*. Substantial sodium and water deficits may occur in patients with diseases affecting predominantly the renal medulla. Renal excretory function in these diseases is usually only moderately impaired.
   The causes of salt-losing nephritis include:
   (i) Medullary cystic disease ('nephronophthisis')
   (ii) Polycystic kidney disease (adult form)
   (iii) Chronic interstitial nephritis
   (iv) Analgesic nephropathy
   (v) Sickle cell disease
   (vi) Partial obstruction
   (vii) Chronic GN (very rare)
3. *Addison's disease*. Typically there is hyperkalaemia and mild pre-renal uraemia in addition to hyponatraemia. Urinary sodium is high but urinary potassium is low (< 20 mmol/l). Random plasma cortisol may be normal if the patient is stressed. An ACTH stimulation test may be required to demonstrate the adrenal insufficiency.
4. *Bicarbonaturia* accompanying proximal renal tubular acidosis (RTA) (see Chapter 6) or metabolic alkalosis causes obligatory losses of cations, mainly sodium and potassium, to maintain electrical neutrality.
5. *Ketonuria*. Ketoacids are a further example of anions whose renal excretion demand obligatory urinary sodium and potassium losses in diabetic or alcoholic ketoacidosis or in starvation.
6. *Osmotic diuretics* cause increased sodium and water excretion by increasing urine flow rates. The principal osmotic diuretics are: glucose in diabetic ketoacidosis or hyperosmolar coma; urea which causes post-obstructive diuresis; and mannitol, usually prescribed for cerebral oedema.

Management of hyponatraemia
Treatment of hyponatraemia depends on the cause; the degree of hyponatraemia present and the severity of symptoms.
1. *Specific causes* should be treated if possible, e.g. replacement of thyroid or adrenocortical hormones, management of hyperglycaemia, diuretics for oedema states, removal of pain, stress, drugs affecting ADH etc.
2. *Water restriction* is appropriate in normal or increased ECF volume causes of hyponatraemia. For water restriction to be effective intake must be restricted to *less* than measured urine output plus an estimate of insensible losses.
3. *Drug therapy* directed at producing nephrogenic diabetes insipidus is useful in chronic SIADH when voluntary water restriction is unsuccessful. Demethylchlortetracycline is the usual agent used. Lithium is a less satisfactory alternative.

The above measures will restore plasma sodium towards normal over a period of several days. If the patient has severe and/or symptomatic hyponatraemia it may be necessary to raise plasma sodium more rapidly. In states of ECF volume depletion rehydration with 0.9% sodium chloride will restore plasma sodium quickly. When ECF volume is increased a combination of hypertonic (e.g. 3%) sodium chloride and frusemide may be used. Renal sodium and chloride losses are replaced as a hypertonic solution thus ensuring net water loss e.g. if a diuresis of 1 l/h is induced and the measured urinary sodium loss can be replaced by 200 ml of 3% sodium chloride, a net water loss of 800 ml will have occurred. The desired net negative water balance can be calculated as follows:

70 kg man. Plasma Na = 115 mmol/l
Total body water (TBW) = Wt 60% = 70 × 0.6 = 42L
Net negative water balance required is:

$$\frac{\text{Desired plasma Na (mmol/l)}}{\text{Actual plasma Na (mmol/l)}} \times \text{TBW}$$

to increase plasma Na to 130 mmol/l = $\frac{130}{115} \times 42 = 47.5$ 1

∴ 47.5 − 42 = 5.51 net negative water balance is needed to raise plasma Na to 130 mmol/l.

HYPERNATRAEMIA

Hypernatraemia is seen less commonly than hyponatraemia. The reason is that the major cause of hypernatraemia, net water loss, is accompanied by thirst. Severe hypernatraemia is thus rare in adults with free access to water and is seen predominantly in the very young, very old, unconscious patients or in the rare patient with disordered thirst regulation.

Symptoms and signs of hypernatraemia

Symptoms
1. Thirst
2. Restlessness
3. Irritability
4. Lethargy
5. Muscle twitching

Signs
1. Depressed sensorium
2. Hyperreflexia
3. Spasticity
4. Focal neurological signs

5. Coma
6. Seizures and death

CNS symptoms predominate. Severe cellular dehydration leads to tearing of intracerebral vessels with subsequent subcortical or subarachnoid haemorrage. Venous sinus thrombosis also occurs.

Diagnosis of hypernatraemia
The main causes of hypernatraemia are:
1. Renal H_2O losses
   a. nephrogenic diabetes insipidus
   b. central diabetes insipidus
   c. partial diabetes insipidus
   d. hypodipsia
2. Renal Na losses
   a. salt-losing nephritis
   b. osmotic diuretics
3. Extrarenal H_2O losses
   a. respiratory insensible losses
   b. dermal e.g. fever, exercise
4. Extrarenal Na losses
   a. diarrhoea in children
   b. excess sweating
5. Endocrine
   a. primary hyperaldosteronism (Conn's syndrome)
   b. Cushing's syndrome
6. Administration of excess Na
   a. hypertonic haemodialysis
   b. $NaHCO_3$ infusion
   c. NaCl tablets

The diagnostic approach to the hypernatraemic patient is outlined in Figure 8. It is convenient to consider the causes of hypernatraemia in terms of their effect on total body sodium.

Hypernatraemia with increased total body sodium
This is very rare. Hypernatraemia resulting from hypertonic haemodialysis or the administration of hypertonic sodium bicarbonate or sodium chloride tablets is usually obvious from the history. Hypernatraemia in Conn's or Cushing's syndromes is rarely severe and is accompanied by hypokalaemic metabolic alkalosis and urinary potassium wasting. Urinary sodium is > 20 mmol in all of these conditions.

Hypernatraemia with normal total body sodium
This occurs principally where there is net water loss.
1. *Renal water losses* include complete or partial central diabetes insipidus (DI) and nephrogenic DI.

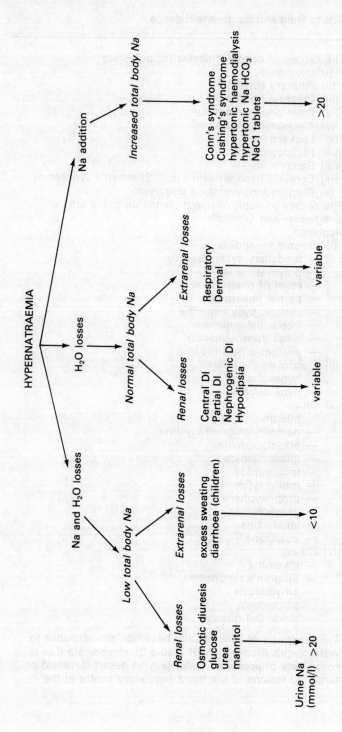

Fig. 8 Diagnostic approach to hypernatraemia

HYPERNATRAEMIA

Na and H₂O losses

H₂O losses

Na addition

Low total body Na

Renal losses
- Osmotic diuresis
- glucose
- urea
- mannitol

Urine Na (mmol/l) >20

Extrarenal losses
- excess sweating
- diarrhoea (children)

<10

Normal total body Na

Renal losses
- Central DI
- Partial DI
- Nephrogenic DI
- Hypodipsia

variable

Extrarenal losses
- Respiratory
- Dermal

variable

Increased total body Na

- Conn's syndrome
- Cushing's syndrome
- hypertonic haemodialysis
- hypertonic Na HCO₃
- NaC1 tablets

>20

a. The causes of central diabetes insipidus are:
   (i) Idiopathic
   (ii) Pituitary surgery
   (iii) Cerebral trauma
   (iv) Brain/pituitary tumour
   (v) Metastatic tumours
   (vi) Leukaemias
   (vii) Histiocytosis X
   (viii) Sarcoidosis
   (ix) Cerebral hypoperfusion (e.g. Sheehan's syndrome)
   (x) Ruptured intracerebral aneurysm
b. The causes of nephrogenic diabetes insipidus are:
   Congenital and familial
   Acquired
   (i) Chronic renal disease
      — medullary cystic disease
      — polycystic disease
      — relief of obstruction
      — partial obstruction
      — chronic pyelonephritis
      — interstitial nephritis
      — renal transplantation
      — analgesic nephropathy
   (ii) Electrolyte disorders
      — hypokalaemia
      — hypercalcaemia
   (iii) Drugs
      — lithium
      — demethylchlortetracycline
      — acetohexamide
      — glibenclamide
      — tolbutamide
      — methoxyflurane
      — propoxyphene
      — amphotericin
      — vinblastine
      — colchicine
   (iv) Others
      — myeloma
      — Sjögren's syndrome
      — amyloidosis
      — sarcoidosis
      — sickle cell disease

The diagnosis of DI is usually based on the response to water deprivation and ADH (Table 3). Hypodipsia due to coma, lack of access to water (e.g. in desert climates) or, rarely, to lesions of the thirst regulatory centre in the

Table 3 Approach to diagnosis in suspected DI

	U_{osm} after dehydration	U_{osm} after ADH
Normal	↑ ↑ ↑	No change
Complete central diabetes insipidus	↓	↑ ↑
Partial central diabetes insipidus	↑	↑ ↑
Nephrogenic diabetes insipidus	↓	↓
Compulsive H_2O drinking	↑ ↑	No change

hypothalamus may also cause hypernatraemia. Urinary osmolality and sodium content are variable in these conditions.

2. *Extra renal water losses* include respiratory losses, e.g. during hyperventilation, and dermal losses, e.g. during fever. These losses may be considerable and are frequently forgotten in assessing fluid requirements, e.g. during fever 500–1000 ml of additional water is lost for every 1°C rise in temperature. Again urinary osmolality and sodium content are variable in these conditions.

Hypernatraemia with low total body sodium
This occurs when both sodium and water are lost, but loss of water predominates.

1. *Renal losses* of sodium and water are principally due to osmotic diuretics. The urine is usually hypotonic and urine sodium is > 20 mmol/l.
2. *Extrarenal losses* of sodium and water causing hypernatraemia include excess sweating, e.g. in marathon runners or hyperpyrexia, and diarrhoea, particularly in children.

Management of hypernatraemia
This depends on the ECF volume status and the rate of development of the hypernatraemia.

1. *ECF volume depletion* should be corrected rapidly with 0.9% sodium chloride to restore plasma volume. Correction of plasma osmolality should thereafter proceed slowly using hypotonic solutions (0.45% sodium chloride or 5% dextrose).
2. *ECF volume expansion* is treated with loop diuretics (e.g. frusemide) to remove excess sodium and water. Dialysis may be necessary if renal failure is present.

3. *Normal ECF volume*. Hypernatraemia in this setting may be corrected by calculating and giving the net water replacement needed to restore plasma sodium. For example, for a 70 kg man with plasma sodium of 160 mmol/l:
   TBW = Wt. 60% = 70 × 0.6 = 42 l

$$\frac{\text{Actual Na (mmol/l)}}{\text{Desired Na (mmol/l)}} \times \text{TBW} = \frac{160}{140} \times 42 = 48 \text{ l}$$

   48 − 42 = 6 l net positive water balance is needed to restore plasma sodium to normal.
   The rate at which plasma sodium should be corrected is important as over rapid correction is liable to cause cerebral oedema. It is recommended that plasma osmolality be corrected at no greater than 2 mosm/hour, preferably over 48 hours or longer.

Normal potassium homeostasis

TOTAL BODY POTASSIUM

Normal total body potassium averages 50 mmol/kg body weight or 3500 mmol for a 70 kg adult. Of this only around 2% is present in the ECF space, the remainder being intracellular. Potassium is thus the predominant intracellular cation with intracellular concentrations of 150 mmol/l compared to normal plasma potassium of 3.5–5 mmol/l. Potassium is important in enzyme function and particularly neuromuscular function.

In clinical practice it is usual to measure plasma potassium which may be a poor indicator of potassium status. Plasma potassium changes substantially in response to a number of variables (see below) without any change in total body potassium. However, in the absence of acid-base or other influences plasma potassium may give a rough guide to total body potassium. In general a reduction of 1 mmol/l in plasma potassium suggests a deficit of 200–300 mmol while an increase of 1 mmol/l suggests a potassium excess of at least 200 mmol. Total body potassium can be measured more directly by whole body counting of ^{40}K or measurement of potassium content of a skeletal muscle biopsy.

FACTORS INFLUENCING PLASMA POTASSIUM

A large number of factors may alter plasma potassium without a change in total body potassium and hence make estimation of potassium status difficult.
1. *Blood pH*. Acidosis promotes potassium egress from cells and hence causes hyperkalaemia even in the presence of normal total body potassium. Alkalosis has the opposite effect on cellular potassium and may cause hypokalaemia. As a rule of thumb a change in plasma potassium of around 0.6 mmol/l is expected for each 0.1 unit pH change, e.g. if normal potassium is 4 mmol/l and pH 7.4 then when blood pH is 7.2 plasma potassium should be no greater than 5.2 mmol/l if acidosis is the only stimulus to hyperkalaemia.

2. *Insulin* promotes potassium entry into cells independently of its effect on glucose transport, explaining in part the hyperkalaemia that may accompany insulin deficiency states such as diabetic ketoacidosis.
3. *Aldosterone* promotes urinary potassium excretion. However, it has been suggested that aldosterone has a wider role in promoting potassium uptake in all cells thus offsetting the tendency to hyperkalaemia that accompanies potassium loading.
4. *Adrenaline* and other β agonists also promote cellular potassium uptake and hence tend to cause hypokalaemia.

MAINTENANCE OF POTASSIUM BALANCE

The dietary intake of potassium in a healthy adult varies from 50 to 150 mmol/24 hours. Over 90% of this daily intake is normally excreted via the kidneys, the primary regulators of external potassium balance. The remainder is excreted in the faeces. Faecal potassium excretion may be a significant source of potassium excretion in patients with advanced renal failure.

Renal potassium excretion
The capacity of the kidneys to vary potassium excretion is extremely large with urinary potassium excretion ranging from a low of 5 mmol/l to a high of over 100 mmol/l in situations of potassium depletion or excess respectively. Under normal circumstances urinary potassium reflects dietary potassium intake and will thus be 50–150 mmol/24 hours. The renal handling of potassium is summarised in Figure 9.
1. *Glomerular filtration.* Potassium is freely filtrated at the glomerulus. If plasma potassium is 4 mmol/l this will generate (assuming normal GFR of 125 ml/min) 720 mmol filtered K^+/24 hours. It is estimated that 10–20% of plasma potassium is protein bound and thus not freely filtrable so that in normal circumstances filtered potassium is around 612 mmol/24 hours.
2. *Proximal tubule.* Up to 70% of filtered potassium is reabsorbed by the proximal tubule, probably by an active transport mechanism that is independent of sodium reabsorption.
3. *Loop of Henle.* Around 20–25% of filtered potassium is reabsorbed in the ascending limb of the loop of Henle. This is probably a passive process occuring down the electrochemical gradient that results from active Cl reabsorption in this segment of the nephron (see p. 6).
4. *Distal tubule* is the site of net potassium secretion. This secretion is mainly a passive process that occurs down the electrochemical gradient generated by the large transepithelial

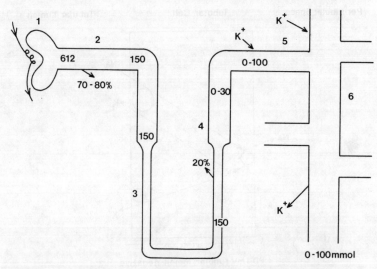

Fig. 9 Renal handling of K⁺. Figures represent absolute amount of potassium (mmol/l) presented in each segment of the nephron. Percentages refer to % reabsorbed at the sites indicate. Net secretion of potassium takes place in the distal tubule and cortical collecting ducts. 1. Glomerulus; 2. Proximal tubule; 3. Thin descending loop of Henle; 4. Thick ascending loop of Henle; 5. Distal tubule; 6. Collecting duct.

potential difference in this segment of the nephron. The gradient is maintained by active sodium-potassium exchange at the basolateral membrane of the tubular cell. This latter mechanism (a Na-K ATPase) is controlled by aldosterone. Distal tubular control of potassium secretion is summarised in Figure 10.

5. *Collecting ducts* have the ability both to reabsorb and secrete potassium. Active potassium secretion has been demonstrated in cortical collecting ducts and is probably under the control of aldosterone. Active net potassium reabsorption occurs in medullary collecting ducts.

FACTORS INFLUENCING POTASSIUM EXCRETION

The major factors that are known or suspected to alter renal potassium excretion are:
1. Aldosterone
2. Acid-base status
   a. acute acidosis—urinary K⁺ ↓
   b. alkalosis—urinary K⁺ ↑
   c. chronic acidosis—urinary K⁺ ↑

Peritubular Space   Tubular Cell   Tubular Lumen

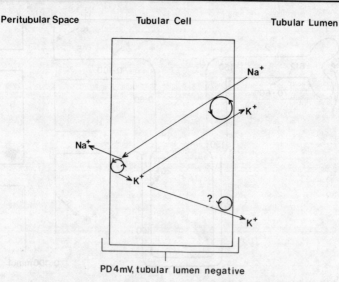

PD 4 mV, tubular lumen negative

Fig. 10 Distal tubular K^+ transport. Intracellular K^+ content is kept high by active transport of K^+ into cells in exchange for Na at the basolateral membrane. Tubular K^+ secretion is mainly passive though some active transport may take place. Na^+ moves passively into the tubular cell from the tubular lumen down its concentration gradient and is extracted actively by the basolateral membrane Na^+–K^+ATPase.

3. Tubular fluid flow rate
4. Na^+ intake
5. K^+ intake
6. Diuretics
   a. K^+ losing
      (i) osmotic (e.g. mannitol, glucose)
      (ii) thiazides
      (iii) carbonic anhydrase inhibitors
      (iv) loop diuretics (e.g. frusemide)
   b. K^+ retaining
      (i) spironolactone
      (ii) triamterene

Aldosterone
Aldosterone has profound effects on sodium and potassium homeostasis. Control of its release is summarised in Figure 5. Adrenal insufficiency causes potassium retention and sodium wasting while mineralocorticoid excess results in sodium retention and potassium wasting with hypokalaemia. Aldosterone

exerts its effects on potassium and sodium excretion mainly in the distal tubule and cortical collecting ducts.

Acid-base status
Renal potassium excretion is profoundly influenced by acid-base status. In acute metabolic or respiratory acidosis, renal potassium excretion is reduced due to displacement of potassium from cells by hydrogen ion and hence reduction in the potassium available for tubular secretion. In metabolic or respiratory alkalosis renal potassium excretion is increased, since the reduced extracellular hydrogen ion concentration drives potassium into renal tubular cells, thus increasing the potassium available for tubular secretion. In chronic metabolic or respiratory acidosis peritubular potassium uptake is enchanced, offsetting the effect of low blood pH on potassium distribution, and renal potassium excretion increases. Substantial potassium deficits may thus be encountered in patients with chronic acidosis.

Tubular fluid flow rate
This directly influences potassium excretion which is higher at high rates of fluid delivery. It is independent of the rate of sodium delivery. The increased potassium excretion is the result of an increase in the concentration gradient favouring potassium secretion and the rapidity with which potassium can be transported to the tubular lumen and washed out by the increased urine flow.

Sodium intake
Sodium loading causes a kaliuresis that is mainly the result of the accompanying increase in tubular fluid flow rate. Increased sodium delivery per se has no effect on potassium excretion. Prolonged sodium restriction is accompanied by reduced urinary potassium due to reduced tubular fluid flow rate and enhanced potassium reabsorption in medullary collecting ducts.

Potassium intake
Under normal circumstances urinary potassium adapts rapidly to changes in dietary potassium due primarily to alterations in peritubular potassium uptake. High potassium diet is associated with enhanced peritubular potassium uptake mediated via the effect of aldosterone on the basolateral membrane sodium-potassium ATPase. Low potassium intake has the opposite effect on peritubular potassium uptake and also enhances medullary collecting duct potassium reabsorption.

Diuretics
Diuretics alter urinary potassium excretion by a variety of mechanisms. Diuretics with a kaliuretic action (osmotic diuretics,

carbonic anhydrase inhibitors, thiazides, loop diuretics) probably all cause increased urinary potassium by increasing tubular fluid flow rate. Inhibition of proximal tubular fluid reabsorption (e.g. metolazone) contributes to kaliuresis by reducing proximal potassium reabsorption. Carbonic anhydrase inhibitors may have a direct effect on distal potassium secretion.

The potassium retaining diuretics spironolactone and triamterene have different modes of action. Spironolactone is a competitive inhibitor of aldosterone and thus produces a state of relative hypoadrenalism with consequent potassium retention and mild natriuresis. Triamterene alters the transluminal electrical potential difference in favour of potassium retention. Both of these agents act predominently on potassium secretion in cortical collecting ducts rather than distal tubules.

Mineralocorticoid drugs
Fludrocortisone, a potent mineralocorticoid, and carbenoxolone, derived from liquorice which contains the mineralocorticoid glycyrrhizinic acid, both resemble aldosterone in producing sodium retention and potassium loss.

Disorders of potassium homeostasis

Since plasma potassium is an unreliable guide to total body potassium but whole body potassium measurements are not practical for routine clinical use, it is not convenient to discuss disorders of potassium homeostasis in terms of change in whole body potassium. Instead it is more useful to consider disorders of potassium homeostasis as disorders of plasma potassium i.e. hypokalaemia or hyperkalaemia.

HYPOKALAEMIA

A wide variety of disorders may give rise to hypokalaemia which may occur with or without potassium deficit. The principal causes of hypokalaemia are:
1. Hypokalaemia without K^+ deficit
   a. Alkalosis
   b. Insulin excess
   c. Athletes
   d. Familial hypokalaemic periodic paralysis
2. Hypokalaemia with K^+ deficit
   a. Poor diet—alcoholism, anorexia nervosa, geophagia
   b. Cellular uptake—e.g. R_x of megaloblastic anaemia
   c. GI loss—vomiting/diarrhoea/laxative abuse; ureterosigmoidostomy/long or obstructed ileal loop/villous adenoma
   d. Urinary loss
      (i) excess mineralocorticoids—1° or 2° hyperaldosteronism; Bartter's syndrome; Cushing's syndrome; ectopic ACTH; liquorice abuse and carbenoxolone; Liddles' syndrome
      (ii) RTA—proximal or distal
           osmotic diuretics
           diuretics
           carbenicillin
           leukaemia

Hypokalaemia without potassium deficit
In these conditions hypokalaemia is due to shift of potassium into cells.
1. *Alkalosis*. Hypokalaemia occurs in both metabolic and respiratory alkalosis as a result of transcellular potassium shifts. Plasma potassium should fall by around 0.6 mmol/l for each 0.1 increase in pH so that some impression of whether there is a true potassium deficit can be had from plasma potassium. Metabolic alkalosis is frequently accompanied by a potassium deficit.
2. *Insulin excess* may cause hypokalaemia by driving potassium into cells. Acute hyperglycaemia may cause hypokalaemia partly through increased insulin release.
3. *Athletes*, particularly distance runners, may have mild hypokalaemia without any evidence of a potassium deficit.
4. *Familial periodic paralysis*. The hypokalaemic variety of this disorder has an autosomal dominant mode of inheritance. Characteristically there are recurrent bouts of flaccid paralysis, accompanied by a fall in plasma potassium to 1–2 mmol/l, resulting from potassium movement into skeletal muscle cells. The aetiology of the potassium flux is unknown.

Hypokalaemia with potassium deficit
Hypokalaemia that cannot be accounted for by transcellular potassium shifts is due to true potassium deficit. The main causes are inadequate potassium intake, gastrointestinal potassium losses and renal potassium losses.

Inadequate potassium intake
This is a significant factor in hypokalaemia in the elderly, infirm and insane. Alcoholism and anorexia nervosa are also accompanied by low potassium intake while geophagia may produce striking potassium losses by binding of potassium to ingested clays. In situations such as hyperalimentation or treatment of megaloblastic anaemia, cellular uptake of potassium may outstrip the dietary supply, with resultant hypokalaemia.

Extra-renal potassium loss
1. *Gastrointestinal*. When potassium loss is extrarenal and of some days duration, effective renal potassium conservation ensures a very low urinary potassium. A urinary potassium of <20 mmol/l should therefore suggest extrarenal potassium loss, usually from the gastrointestinal tract. Substantial potassium losses usually occur from the lower gastrointestinal tract, e.g. in diarrhoea, villous adenoma of the rectum or a small bowel fistula. Chronic laxative abuse may be less obvious. Prolonged vomiting or nasogastric suction may also cause hypokalaemia in association with metabolic alkalosis. Lower gastrointestinal tract potassium losses will also be accompanied by metabolic

alkalosis unless large amounts of bicarbonate are also being lost.

2. *Hyperhidrosis* may rarely cause extrarenal potassium depletion.

Urinary potassium loss
A urinary potassium >20 mmol/l indicates that the kidneys are the primary site of potassium loss. Renal hypokalaemia can be classified according to the underlying acid-base disturbance.

1. Hypokalaemia with metabolic acidosis is seen in diabetic ketoacidosis, proximal and distal renal tubular acidosis (RTA) and during therapy with carbonic anhydrase inhibitors (e.g. acetazolamide; 'Diamox').
2. Hypokalaemia with metabolic alkalosis is the commonest finding in renal potassium wasting states. These conditions may be further subclassified according to urine chloride (Fig. 11):
   a. *Chloride depletion* resulting from chronic upper gastrointestinal loss, diuretics or rarely chloride losing diarrhoea may cause hypokalaemic metabolic alkalosis. Abrupt relief of chronic hypercapnia may also be followed by severe hypokalaemic metabolic alkalosis unless the accompanying chloride deficit is corrected.
   b. *High urinary chloride* and hypokalaemia is encountered in a number of situations such as continued diuretic therapy, Bartter's syndrome and severe potassium depletion (potassium losses in excess of 1000 mmol). Bartter's syndrome is characterised by hypokalaemic metabolic alkalosis, hypereninaemic hyperaldosteronism, normotension and high urinary prostaglandins. This condition may result from a defect in chloride transport in the ascending limb of the loop of Henle.

In all conditions due to excess mineralocorticoid activity there is some degree of hypertension. The causes are shown in Figure 11. Liddle's syndrome is characterised by hypertension, hyporeninaemic hypoaldosteronism and hypokalaemia. It may be due to an as yet unidentified mineralocorticoid. Excess DOC (deoxycorticosterone) is seen in patients with congenital adrenal 11β and 17α-hydroxylase deficiencies.

Clinical features of hypokalaemia
The main clinical features of hypokalaemia are:
1. Cardiac
   a. risk of digoxin toxicity
   b. ECG changes
   c. atrial/ventricular ectopics
   d. cardiac necrosis

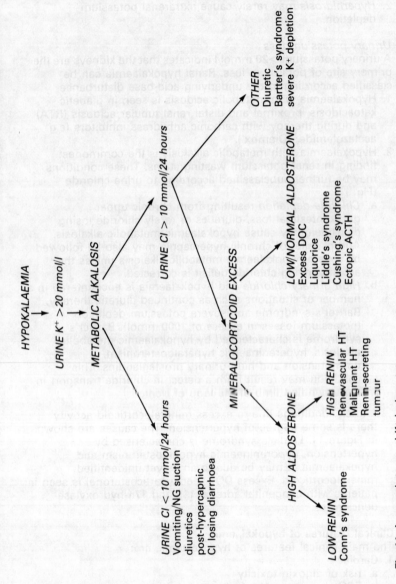

Fig. 11 Approach to renal K⁺ losing states.

HYPOKALAEMIA

URINE K⁺ > 20 mmol/l

METABOLIC ALKALOSIS

URINE Cl < 10 mmol/24 hours
Vomiting/NG suction
diuretics
post-hypercapnic
Cl losing diarrhoea

URINE Cl > 10 mmol/24 hours

MINERALOCORTICOID EXCESS

LOW/NORMAL ALDOSTERONE
Excess DOC
Liquorice
Liddle's syndrome
Cushing's syndrome
Ectopic ACTH

HIGH ALDOSTERONE

LOW RENIN
Conn's syndrome

HIGH RENIN
Renovascular HT
Malignant HT
Renin-secreting
tumour

OTHER
Diuretic
Bartter's syndrome
severe K⁺ depletion

2. Neuromuscular
   a. gastrointestinal—constipation, ileus
   b. striated—weakness, paralysis
   c. acute rhabdomyolysis
3. Renal
   a. reversible ↓ in GFR
   b. polyuria/polydipsia
   c. Na$^+$ retention
   d. Hyponatraemia
   e. Cl wasting
   f. metabolic alkalosis
4. Endocrine
   a. ↓ aldosterone
   b. ↑ renin
   c. ↓ prostaglandins
   d. ↑ insulin

The majority of symptoms and signs reflect impaired
neuromuscular function.

1. *Cardiac* manifestations are the most important. Acute effects
   include atrial and ventricular ectopics and, more importantly, a
   predisposition to fatal ventricular arrhythmias during
   concomitant digoxin therapy. Cardiac necrosis and myocardial
   fibrosis may accompany chronic hypokalaemia. ECG changes
   in hypokalaemia are shown in Figure 12.
2. *Neuromuscular* symptoms occur at plasma potassium
   <3.0 mmol/l. Muscle weakness may be severe enough to cause
   respiratory insufficiency. Acute rhabdomyolysis is rare.
3. *Renal* effects of low potassium are seen mainly with chronic
   hypokalaemia. The reduction in GFR is reversible but
   polyuria/polydipsia which reflect a renal concentrating defect
   (diminished renal response to ADH) may persist due to
   interstitial fibrosis with permanent tubular damage.
4. *Endocrine* changes associated with hypokalaemia are mainly a
   reflection of the physiological response to potassium
   depletion; thus aldosterone may be low and renin elevated.
   Severe potassium depletion interferes directly with pancreatic
   insulin release and may result in frank glucose intolerance.

Management of hypokalaemia
This depends on the cause. In hypokalaemia without potassium
deficit potassium replacement is unnecessary and treatment
directed at the underlying cause will correct plasma potassium.
However, in hypokalaemia due to metabolic alkalosis some
potassium supplementation is usually required.

For hypokalaemia with potassium deficit the treatment depends
on the severity of hypokalaemia, the magnitude of the potassium
deficit and the symptoms, if any. The potassium deficit can be

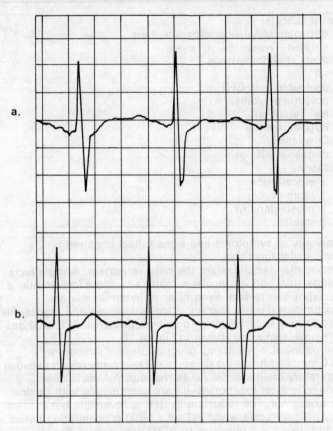

Fig. 12 ECG changes in hypokalaemia. (a) Lead V_3. Serum K^+ 1.8 mmol/l.
Note the small inverted P wave. The PR interval is 0.08 s. The T wave is
small and there is a prominent U wave giving the appearance of a
prolonged QT interval.
(b) Lead V_3. Serum K^+ 2.8 mmol/l. The P wave is now normal with a
normal PR interval (0.14 s). The T wave is now of normal amplitude and
the U wave less prominent.

estimated from the plasma potassium (see p. 27): a fall of
1 mmol/l approximates to a potassium deficit of 200–300 mmol.

In general oral potassium replacement is desirable unless the
patient is paralysed, comatose or on digoxin when I.V.
replacement should be used. For a mild deficit (<500 mmol)
replacement at 40 mmol/24 hours is adequate. For larger deficits
oral or I.V. administration of 80–120 mmol/24 hours is required.

Oral potassium may be given as enteric coated tablets (Slow K, Ciba = 8 mmol/tab) or effervescent tablets (Sando K, Sandoz = 12 mmol/tab). Oral potassium preparations may cause gastrointestinal upset and enteric coated tablets are reported to cause small bowel ulceration. New microencapsulated preparations of potassium salts may produce less gastrointestinal upset.

For patients on diuretic therapy routine potassium supplementation is not needed unless potassium falls below 3 mmol/l. In this situation oral potassium supplements may be used or, more logically, a potassium retaining agent such as triamterene or spironolactone. Potassium retaining diuretics should be used with extreme caution in patients with renal impairment.

HYPERKALAEMIA

Hyperkalaemia may occur in a wide variety of clinical settings though dangerous hyperkalaemia is seen most frequently in renal failure. The main causes of hyperkalaemia are:

1. Pseudohyperkalaemia
   a. tourniquet
   b. haemolysed sample
   c. thrombocytosis/leukocytosis
2. Redistribution
   a. acidosis
   b. glucose loading in diabetics
   c. β blockers
   d. familial hyperkalaemic periodic paralysis
   e. succinylcholine
   f. arginine HCl
   g. digoxin overdosage
3. Potassium excess
   a. Diminished excretion
      (i) acute/chronic renal failure
      (ii) K⁺sparing diuretics
      (iii) mineralocorticoid deficiency
      — Addison's disease
      — hyporeninaemic hypoaldosteronism
      — NSAIDs e.g. indomethacin
      (iv) selective impairment of renal K⁺ secretion, SLE, renal transplant, sickle cell disease, myeloma, amyloid, cyclosporin A
   b. Excess input of K⁺
      (i) haemolysis, rhabdomyolysis, burns
      (ii) salt substitutes, diet, K⁺ salts of penicillins

Pseudohyperkalaemia

When serum potassium is found to be high it is important to be sure that this reflects true hyperkalaemia. Spurious elevations in serum potassium are seen when blood is collected after prolonged application of a tourniquet or when the sample is haemolysed. Severe thrombocytosis or leukocytosis may increase serum potassium due to release of potassium from the cells during clotting. In these circumstances plasma potassium, measured in a heparinized sample, will be normal.

Redistribution

Redistribution of potassium between the ICF and ECF spaces is an important cause of hyperkalaemia.

1. *Metabolic or respiratory acidosis* increases plasma potassium causing potassium egress from cells. There may be some accompanying potassium excess e.g. in chronic renal failure.
2. *Glucose loading* in normal subjects causes potassium to fall but in diabetics plasma potassium may rise due to insulin deficiency.
3. *β blockers* can cause hyperkalaemia by preventing potassium entry into cells. Dangerous hyperkalaemia as a result of β blockade alone is very rare.
4. *Familial hyperkalaemic periodic paralysis* is a rare autosomal dominant condition characterized by episodes of hyperkalaemic paralysis, lasting around 1 hour, in response to stress, exercise, cold exposure or hunger.
5. *Succinylcholine* also promotes potassium egress from cells and is particularly dangerous in patients with renal failure undergoing surgery.
6. *Arginine HCl* and other cationic amino acids also cause hyperkalaemia by promoting potassium egress from cells
7. *Digoxin overdosage* may rarely cause hyperkalaemia by interfering with membrane sodium-potassium ATPase.

Potassium excess

Diminished potassium excretion

Reduction in potassium excretion usually indicates difficulty with renal potassium secretion as the kidneys are the major route of potassium excretion (see p. 28).

1. *Acute and chronic renal failure* may both be accompanied by hyperkalaemia particularly when GFR is <10 ml/min. Severe hyperkalaemia in patients with GFR >15–20 ml/min is usually due to some additional factor such as systemic acidosis, the use of potassium sparing diuretics or ingestion of a high potassium diet.

2. Potassium sparing diuretics produce hyperkalaemia by inhibition of aldosterone (spironolactone) or by blocking aldosterone-independent renal potassium secretion (triamterene and amiloride).
3. *Mineralocorticoid deficiency* is accompanied by hyperkalaemia often with hyperchloraemic acidosis. It may be due to adrenocortical insufficiency (Addison's disease), hyporeninaemic hypoaldosteronism or to administration of NSAIDs such as indomethacin. Hyporeninaemic hypoaldosteronism is being recognised with increasing frequency in diabetes and interstitial nephritis.
4. Selective impairment of renal potassium secretion is seen in a variety of conditions such as SLE, renal transplantation, sickle cell disease, myeloma, amyloid and cyclosporin A nephrotoxicity.

Excess input of potassium
1. *Endogenous potassium* excesses result from acute intravascular haemolysis (e.g. mis-matched transfusion), acute rhabdomyolysis or extensive burns. Any catabolic state may produce hyperkalaemia when there is associated renal failure.
2. *Exogenous potassium* excesses result from ingestion of potassium containing salt substitutes, potassium salts of penicillins or a diet rich in potassium. All of these are more likely to precipitate dangerous hyperkalaemia in patients with chronic renal failure.

Clinical features of hyperkalaemia
The main clinical effects of hyperkalaemia are on the cardiac conducting system. Hyperkalaemia produces progressive ECG changes that culminate in cardiac arrest. These changes are summarised in Figure 13.

Symptoms of hyperkalaemia occur late, when plasma potassium is generally >8 mmol/l and cardiotoxicity well advanced. Neuromuscular symptoms such as paraesthesiae, muscle weakness and flaccid paralysis predominate. Nausea, vomiting, abdominal pain and paralytic ileus may also occur.

Treatment of hyperkalaemia
This depends on the cause and severity of the hyperkalaemia. Where hyperkalaemia is due to transcellular shift of potassium, e.g. in acidosis, therapy should be directed towards the underlying cause. Where there is a total body potassium excess it may be necessary to induce a temporary shift of potassium into cells to diminish the risk of cardiac arrest while appropriate therapy for the underlying cause, e.g. renal failure, is instituted.

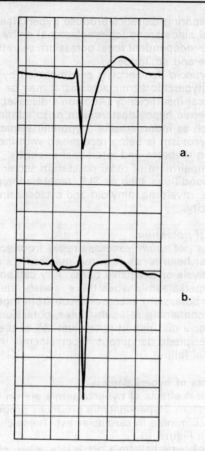

Fig. 13 ECG changes in hyperkalaemia. (a) Lead V₃. Serum K⁺ 7.4 mmol/l.
The P wave is absent and the QRS complex prolonged (0.18 s). The QRS
blends into the T wave which is less prominent than is usual in
hyperkalaemia.
(b) Lead V₃. Serum K⁺ 5.7 mmol/l. The P wave has returned and the PR
interval is at the upper limit of normal. The QRS complex is now of
normal duration.

Acute hyperkalaemia

The management of life-threatening acute hyperkalaemia is
outlined in Table 4. Immediate management consists of
administration of I.V. Ca gluconate 10–30 ml 10% and Na HCO₃
50–150 mmol followed by the I.V. infusion of 50 g glucose
(100 ml of 50%) and 10 units soluble insulin over 15–30 minutes.

Table 4 Management of life-threatening hyperkalaemia

	Treatment	Mode of action
Immediate (few mins)	10–30 ml 10% Ca gluconate I.V. 50–150 mmol Na HCO_3 I.V.	antagonises membrane effects of K^+ excess moves K^+ into cells
Intermediate (15–30 mins)	infuse 50 g glucose and 10 u soluble insulin I.V.	moves K^+ into cells
Long-term (60 mins)	give cation exchange resin 30–60 g rectally or 30 g orally	removes K^+ from body
Haemodialysis/peritoneal dialysis. Used only in renal failure. Effective within a few minutes of starting therapy		removes K^+ from body

These manoeuvres serve to protect the myocardium and induce movement of potassium into cells.

Removal of excess potassium can be achieved by the oral or rectal administration of a cationic exchange resin such as Ca^{++} Resonium or Resonium A. Haemodialysis or peritoneal dialysis are effective means of removing substantial amounts of potassium but are used mainly in renal failure.

Chronic hyperkalaemia
Ideally this should be managed by removing the cause. Chronic administration of a cation exchange resin such as Ca Resonium may be required. Na^+ containing resins (e.g. Resonium A) are best avoided in renal failure as they may produce sodium and water retention. Mineralocorticoids, e.g. fludrocortisone, should be used in Addison's disease and hyporeninaemic hypoaldosteronism. Diuretics, e.g. frusemide, may also reduce hyperkalaemia in hyporeninaemic hypoaldosteronism. Dietary potassium restriction is appropriate in situations where the tendency to hyperkalaemia cannot be satisfactorily treated e.g. chronic renal failure.

Normal acid-base homeostasis

The blood pH of a healthy individual is in the range 7.35–7.45. Such tight control of blood pH is essential for normal metabolic functions including enzyme activity, blood clotting and neuromuscular activity. Extremes of blood pH in the range 6.8–8.0 are fatal unless corrected very rapidly.

DEFINITIONS

In order to understand acid-base homeostasis some brief explanation and definition of the terms used is required. An *acid* is a substance that can dissociate to yield hydrogen ions. A *base* is a substance which can accept hydrogen ions. *Strong acids* such as hydrochloric acid are completely dissociated in aqueous solution, whereas *weak acids* such as carbonic acid are only partially dissociated in aqueous solution. The extent to which weak acids (or bases) dissociate depends on the dissociation constant (pK) for that acid (or base).

Buffering is the reaction to a change in hydrogen ion concentration by any weak acids or bases present. This reaction minimises the change in pH either by binding part of an addition of hydrogen ion or by dissociating further to replenish a fall in hydrogen ion.

e.g. $\quad H^+ + Cl^- + Na^+HCO_3 \quad \rightarrow \quad H_2CO_3 + Na^+Cl^- \quad\quad$ (1)
$\quad\quad$ strong acid $\quad$ buffer $\quad\quad\quad\quad\quad$ weak acid $\quad$ neutral salt

Conventially the acidity/alkalinity of biological fluids is given as pH. This term is derived from the hydrogen ion concentration. In blood, pH is derived from the relationship between hydrogen ion concentration and carbonic acid. This may be more clearly understood if the dissociation constant, K, for this weak acid is studied:

$$[H_2CO_3] \rightleftharpoons [H^+] + [HCO_3]$$

$$K = [H^+] \frac{[HCO_3^-]}{[HCO_3^-]}$$

$$\therefore [H^+] = K \frac{[HCO_3^-]}{[HCO_3^-]} \tag{2}$$

$$\therefore \log H^+ = \log K + \log \frac{[HCO_3^-]}{[HCO_3^-]}$$

Since $pH = -\log_{10}[H^+]$

$$pH = pK + \log_{10}\frac{[HCO_3^-]}{[HCO_3^-]} \quad \text{(Henderson Hasselbalch Equation)}$$

$$= 6.1 + \log_{10}\frac{[HCO_3^-]}{[HCO_3^-]}$$

The concentration of carbonic acid $[H_2CO_3]$ depends upon the amount of carbon dioxide present in the blood (Pa_{CO_2}). In fact when measured in mmHg $[H_2CO_3]$ is 0.03 Pa_{CO_2}

$$\therefore pH = 6.1 + \log_{10}\frac{[HCO_3^-]}{0.03 Pa_{CO_2}} \tag{3}$$

The Henderson-Hasselbalch equation is used in analysis of acid-base disorders. Measurement of any two parameters (usually pH and Pa_{CO_2}) allows the third to be calculated.

THREATS TO pH

There are two major threats to pH which must be overcome:
1. *Volatile acid.* Between 13000 and 20000 mmol of carbon dioxide is produced daily by oxidative metabolism. Hydration of this carbon dioxide yields hydrogen ion as follows:

$$CO_2 + H_2O \rightleftharpoons H_2CO_3 \rightleftharpoons HCO_3^- + H^+$$

This occurs spontaneously and also under the influence of carbonic anhydrase. Since carbon dioxide is under normal circumstances blown off by the lungs, the reactions in equation 4 are driven to the left and hydrogen ion generation is minimised. Indeed the efficiency of the lungs in removing carbon dioxide at a rate of 10–15 mmol/min may be contrasted with the ability of the kidneys to secrete only 0.4 mmol/min of H^+ under conditions of maximal H^+ excretion.

2. *Fixed acids*. Metabolism of dietary protein yields about 1 mmol of strong acid (i.e. H^+)/kg body weight. H^+ itself cannot be eliminated by respiration, but it is immediately buffered by anionic groups of proteins and inorganic phosphate and, most of all, by the large body store of HCO_3^- (see below), so that the actual change in pH is minimised. Steady state is achieved, however, by the fact that renal excretion of H^+ matches fixed acid production.

BUFFER SYSTEMS

Providing that respiratory function is adequate the relatively massive production of volatile acid poses little long-term threat to pH as the carbon dioxide produced by oxidative metabolism is blown off by the lungs. However short-term buffering of the hydrogen ion associated with volatile acid production is required to prevent a disastrous fall in pH. Fixed acid production is more problematic since the acids produced are largely strong acids and their slower renal excretion needs longer-term buffering. There are thus two major types of buffer: short-term buffers which have a restricted capacity but can buffer an acid-load within seconds or minutes, e.g. the plasma bicarbonate buffer system; and longer-term buffers which can buffer an acid load over a period of hours rather than seconds, e.g. tissue proteins.

Fast buffering
This acts as an immediate brake on the fall in pH that results from an acid load. These buffers are largely within the blood.

The bicarbonate buffer system
This system accounts for the buffering of around 40% of an acid load via buffering in blood and interstitial fluid. The general equation for the activity of the bicarbonate buffer system is:

$$H^+ + Cl^- + Na^+ + HCO_3^- \rightleftharpoons Na^+ + Cl^- + H_2CO_3 \qquad (1)$$

However, H_2CO_3 dissociates to $CO_2 + H_2O$. Since the carbon dioxide is normally blown off by the lungs the reactions are pulled to the right minimising may change in hydrogen ion concentration and hence pH. Note that a bicarbonate ion is used up in buffering the hydrogen ion. The main limiting factor in the bicarbonate buffer system is the capacity to regenerate bicarbonate.

Plasma inorganic phosphate and plasma proteins
These can together rapidly buffer around 2% of an acid load:

e.g. $H^+ + Pr^- \rightleftharpoons HPr$
and $H^+ + HPO_4^- \rightleftharpoons H_2PO_4$

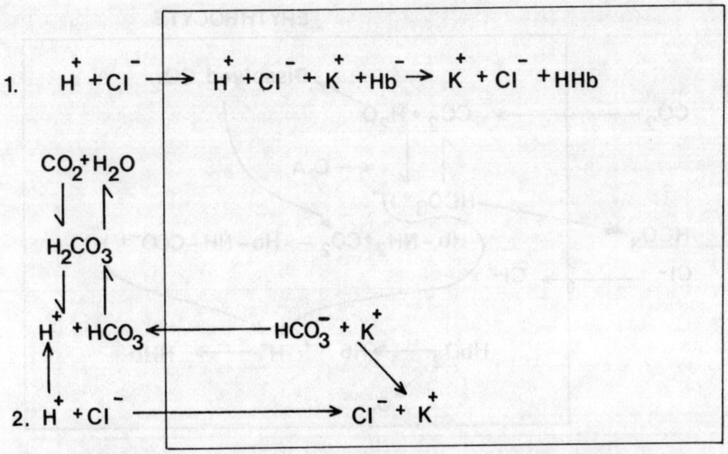

Fig. 14 Buffering of fixed acid by erythrocytes. Erythrocytes may buffer fixed acid in two ways. (1) Hydrogen ion may be buffered directly by haemoglobin. (2) The anion of a strong acid (e.g. HCl) may enter the erythrocyte in exchange for bicarbonate. The bicarbonate buffers excess hydrogen ion and is converted to carbon dioxide which can then be lost via the lungs.

Red blood cells

These cells can act as a rapid buffer system via the carbamate reaction of haemoglobin. Erythrocytes are also freely permeable to carbon dioxide so that both fixed and volatile acids may be buffered by haemoglobin. For fixed acids, buffering in erythrocytes proceeds as shown in Figure 14.

The carbamate reaction (Fig. 15) is a method for the rapid buffering of volatile acid. A secondary, though no less important, function is that carbamation of haemoglobin in capillaries prevents the *rise* in pH that would normally result from deoxygenation of haemoglobin. (Haemoglobin, like many proteins is negatively charged. Oxyhaemoglobin and deoxyhaemoglobin each have a different pK with deoxyhaemoglobin being more basic and thus tending to make pH rise.)

Slow buffering

This will absorb the major component of a fixed acid load (some 60%) for later renal excretion. The major long-term buffers are tissue proteins, intracellular organic phosphates and bone phosphates.

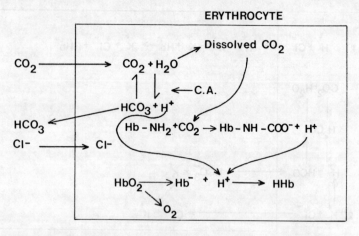

Fig. 15 The carbamate reaction in erythrocytes. C.A. = carbonic anhydrase. Erythrocytes are freely permeable to CO_2 and have plentiful carbonic anhydrase. Hydrogen ion is therefore generated in response to influx of CO_2 into erythrocytes. Bicarbonate produced by carbonic anhydrase activity leaves the erythrocyte in exchange for chloride and can buffer hydrogen ion in plasma. The hydrogen ion in turn is buffered by haemoglobin. This is also important in preventing the rise in pH that would normally accompany deoxygenation of haemoglobin (deoxy haemoglobin has a higher pK^1 than oxyhaemoglobin). Formation of carbamino-haemoglobin (the carbamate reacation) is central to the removal of CO_2 in venous blood. The CO_2 is liberated and blown off in the lungs.

RENAL HANDLING OF HYDROGEN ION

It is apparent from the above that the operation of the bicarbonate buffer system in particular would lead to rapid exhaustion of buffering capacity unless the buffer were somehow replenished. In addition, the hydrogen ion associated with buffered fixed acid must be excreted. The kidneys play a vital role in both the regeneration of bicarbonate buffer and in excretion of fixed acid.

Bicarbonate 'reabsorption'

Normally 80–90% of filtered bicarbonate is 'reabsorbed' by the end of the proximal tubule, the remainder being 'reabsorbed' at more distal sites. Bicarbonate 'reabsorption' is under the influence of carbonic anhydrase. (Fig. 16) which is present in both renal tubular cells and on the luminal surface of tubular cells. As can be seen from Figure 16 bicarbonate is not reabsorbed directly but is regenerated from hydration of carbon

BLOOD   TUBULAR CELL   URINE

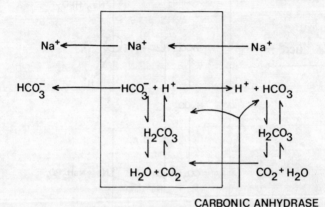

CARBONIC ANHYDRASE

Fig. 16 Renal bicarbonate reabsorption. Carbonic anhydrase within tubular cells and on the luminal brush border promotes 'reabsorption' of bicarbonate. Inhibition of carbonic anhydrase reduces bicarbonate 'reabsorption' resulting in a normal anion-gap type metabolic acidosis.

dioxide within renal tubular cells. Note that bicarbonate 'reabsorption' is closely linked to active sodium reabsorption and hydrogen ion excretion. Note too that the excreted hydrogen ion is also generated within the tubular cell during hydration of carbon dioxide so that no net acid excretion occurs. Fixed acid cannot be excreted by participation in bicarbonate reabsorption.

Excretion of fixed acid
The reabsorption of bicarbonate does not replenish buffer that has been used up in buffering fixed acids. However, net excretion of fixed acid does achieve *new* bicarbonate generation as described below.

Excretion of titratable acidity
This is one means whereby fixed acid can be excreted with net bicarbonate generation as illustrated in Figure 17. Though of minor importance in plasma, buffering by HPO_4^- in urine is quite important, since the concentration is sufficient to buffer substantial amounts of H^+. How much this is can be found by titration to pH 7.4 with strong base, which reverses the buffer

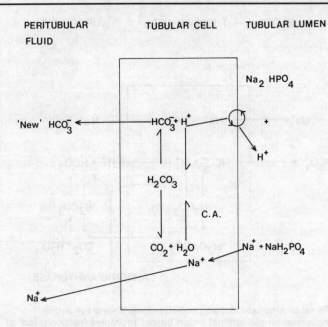

Fig. 17 Excretion of titratable acidity. The excretion of H^+ is also largely dependent on carbonic anhydrase (C.A.) for hydrogen ion production. Excretion of hydrogen ion is active. Sodium movement into the peritubular fluid is also active. Most of the carbon dioxide utilised in hydrogen ion generation is absorbed from the tubular lumen.

reaction. This component of urinary H^+ output has therefore been termed 'titratable acidity'. This term is perhaps not very useful because titration to pH 7.4 does not measure ammonium secretion.

Excretion of ammonium

This is also accompanied by net acid excretion and generation of new bicarbonate. Ammonium is produced in renal tubular cells by deamination of glutamine and other amino acids. The mechanism of ammonium secretion and net bicarbonate gain is illustrated in Figure 18.

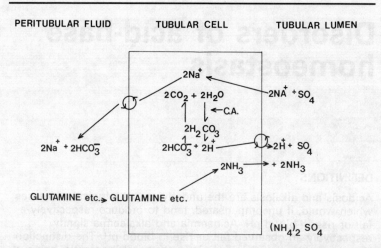

Fig. 18 Renal excretion of ammonium. Glutamine and other amino acids are absorbed via the peritubular fluid and deaminated to form ammonia. Ammonia diffuses passively into the tubular lumen where it is converted into ammonium by the addition of hydrogen ion derived from C.A. activity within the cell. Ammonium is non-reabsorbable and is therefore excreted. At the same time sodium is reabsorbed to maintain electrical neutrality and is pumped actively to the peritubular fluid along with 'new' bicarbonate derived from C.A. activity.

Disorders of acid-base homeostasis

DEFINITIONS

Acidosis and alkalosis are the underlying pathological processes which would, if uncompensated, tend to produce respectively a fall or rise in blood pH. Acidaemia and alkalaemia signify respectively an observed fall or rise in blood pH. The distinction between acidosis and acidaemia is not purely semantic, being of particular significance in mixed acid-base disorders where over- or undercompensation may result in an unexpected blood pH.

ACID-BASE DISORDERS

These may be characterized in several ways. A simple and convenient way of approaching such disorders is in terms of the change in plasma bicarbonate. Renal or respiratory compensatory mechanisms may restore blood pH to near normal so that the primary acid-base disturbance is detectable only by the observed change in plasma bicarbonate.

LOW PLASMA BICARBONATE

This is characteristic of both metabolic acidosis and respiratory alkalosis. These conditions may be distinguished by measuring blood pH which will be reduced in simple metabolic acidosis and increased in simple respiratory alkalosis.

Metabolic acidosis and anion gap

Metabolic acidosis is characterised by a reduced plasma bicarbonate and a variable degree of acidaemia. Final blood pH depends on the nature and severity of the initiating process, rapidity of onset and duration of acidosis. There is a wide range of causes which may be further subdivided into those associated with a normal or increased unmeasured anion gap:

Normal anion gap
1. Bicarbonate loss
   a. diarrhoea

   b. biliary/pancreatic losses
   c. ureterosigmoidostomy
   d. long or obstructed ileal loop bladder
   e. carbonic anhydrase inhibitors
2. Renal tubular dysfunction
   a. distal RTA
   b. proximal RTA
   c. tubulointerstitial disease
3. Addition of acid
   a. ammonium chloride
   b. arginine hydrochloride
   c. lysine hydrochloride

Increased anion gap
1. Overproduction of acid
   a. lactic acidosis
   b. diabetic ketoacidosis
   c. starvation
   d. alcoholic ketoacidosis
   e. salicylates
   f. methanol
   g. ethylene glycol
   h. paraldehyde
2. Renal failure
   a. acute
   b. chronic

The anion gap is the difference between the plasma concentrations of cations and anions and is calculated by subtracting the sum of serum bicarbonate and chloride concentrations from the serum sodium concentration. Normally the result obtained is within the range 8–16 mmol/l.

Calculation of the serum anion gap can be very helpful in the differential diagnosis of acid-base disorders provided care is taken in its interpretation. The normal unmeasured anion gap of 8–16 mmol/l is composed largely of anionic plasma proteins, mainly albumin. Hypoalbuminaemia will therefore reduce the anion gap as may accumulation of cationic proteins such as in myeloma. Indeed a reduced anion gap may be a clue to such disorders and an indication to measure the plasma proteins. The importance of this concept in the interpretation of acid-base disorders is that a 'normal' anion gap in a patient known to be hypoalbuminaemic may still represent significant accumulation of unmeasured anions. If for example the anion gap was 4 mmol in a patient with hypoalbuminaemia the development of, for example, lactic acidosis with the accumulation of 8 mmol/l of lactate, would result in a 'normal' anion gap of 12 mmol/l despite severe metabolic acidosis.

One further situation in which the anion gap may be misleading is in halide poisoning. Bromide and iodine are measured as chloride by most autoanalysers unless specific measures are taken to detect them. However 5 mmol bromide is measured as around 8 mmol of chloride. Thus a patient with unsuspected bromide poisoning and lactic acidosis from the accompanying hypotension might have a 'normal' anion gap. Despite these reservations calculation of the anion gap remains a useful method of separating the different forms of metabolic acidosis.

Metabolic acidosis with normal unmeasured anion gap
This type of metabolic acidosis is seen in association with bicarbonate loss, renal tubular dysfunction or acid loading.
1. *Bicarbonate loss* occurs principally from the gastrointestinal tract as a result of diarrhoea or the loss of pancreatic or biliary secretions, e.g. after biliary tract surgery. A similar hyperchloraemic metabolic acidosis may also be seen following ureterosigmoidostomy or in long or obstructed ileal loop bladders, as the result of intestinal absorption of urinary chloride in exchange for bicarbonate. The metabolic acidosis which accompanies the use of carbonic anhydrase inhibitors e.g. acetazolamide is also of the bicarbonate losing type (see Fig. 16).
2. *Renal tubular dysfunction* may cause metabolic acidosis in a variety of ways. Renal tubular acidosis (RTA) has two major forms:
   a. *Distal RTA* (classical; Type 1; gradient limited) is characterised by acidosis, hypokalaemia and a urinary pH >5.5 irrespective of the degree of acidaemia. The basic defect in distal RTA is the inability of cortical collecting ducts to maintain a high transepithelial hydrogen ion concentration thus impairing net acid excretion. Distal RTA may be primary or acquired and accounts for the vast majority of cases of RTA. The major causes of distal RTA are:
      (i) Primary (idiopathic)
         — Hereditary
         — Sporadic
      (ii) Secondary
         — Dysproteinaemias
            multiple myeloma
            Waldenstrom's macroglobulinaemia
            amyloid
            light-chain disease
            hyperglobulinaemia
         — Tubulo-interstitial disease
            renal transplant
            medullary sponge kidney

                    sickle cell disease
                    hydronephrosis
              — Drugs/toxins
                    amphotericin
                    toluene (glue/paint sniffing)
                    lithium
                    hypercalcaemia
    b. *Proximal RTA* (Type 2; bicarbonate—wasting) is
       characterised by diminished reclamation of bicarbonate by
       the proximal tubule. There is in effect a reduced threshold
       for renal bicarbonate reabsorption. Plasma bicarbonate falls
       until the new threshold value is reached when no further
       bicarbonate loss occurs. Since distal acidification is normal
       patients with proximal RTA may have a low urine pH (5.5)
       along with systemic acidosis. Proximal RTA is usually
       accompanied by other evidence of proximal tubular
       dysfunction such as glycosuria, aminoaciduria,
       phosphaturia, uricosuria and tubular proteinuria (Fanconi
       syndrome). The principal causes of proximal RTA are:
       (i) Primary
       (ii) Secondary
              — Inborn errors of metabolism
                    galactosaemia
                    glycogenosis Type 1
                    hereditary fructose intolerance
                    cystinosis
              — Drugs/toxins
                    heavy metals (Cd,Cu,Hg,Pb)
                    outdate tetracycline
                    6-mercaptopurine
                    carbonic anhydrase inhibitors
                    streptozotocin
              — Dysproteinaemias
                    multiple myeloma
                    amyloid
                    Sjogren's syndrome
                    nephrotic syndrome
              — Other
                    renal transplantation
                    hyperparathyroidism
                    hypervitaminosis D
    c. *Tubulointerstitial diseases* such as analgesic nephropathy
       and chronic interstitial nephritis impair renal tubular
       function more than they reduce GFR. Typically there is
       reduced urinary concentrating ability and an acquired form
       of distal RTA. Hyporeninaemic hypoaldosteronism, e.g. in
       diabetes, has been increasingly recognised as a cause of
       mild hyperchloraemic acidosis accompanied by

hyperkalaemia. This has been termed Type IV RTA but is probably a variant form of distal RTA caused by excessive distal tubular permeability to chloride.

3. *Acid loading* such as the administration of large amounts of ammonium chloride will result in metabolic acidosis. A more subtle cause is administration of cationic amino acids such as lysine and arginine in some parenteral feeding regimes.

Metabolic acidosis with an increased unmeasured anion gap
Increased anion gap type metabolic acidosis may be due to overproduction of organic acid or diminished acid elimination.

1. *Overproduction of acid*
   a. *Lactic acidosis* is a major cause of severe metabolic acidosis. It occurs in a wide range of clinical settings such as severe hypoxia (from shock, low cardiac output or severe anaemia), alcohol intoxication, bigaunides (especially phenformin) or diabetes mellitus. The main pathogenetic mechanism is impaired oxidative metabolism leading to accumulation of excess lactate. Since lactate is normally metabolised in the liver to bicarbonate, hepatic dysfunction may significantly worsen the acid-base disturbance. Lactic acidosis can be diagnosed with certainty only from a measured increase in serum lactate though a presumptive diagnosis can often be made in appropriate clinical situations where other causes of increased anion gap metabolic acidosis have been eliminated.
   b. *Diabetic ketoacidosis* results from overproduction of the organic anions acetoacetate and β hydroxybutyrate in response to insulin deficiency. The diagnosis is usually obvious from the clinical setting and the accompanying hyperglycaemia. The serum nitroprusside (Acetest) reaction is usually positive in ketoacidosis. This test measures acetoacetate so that in conditions where β hydroxybutyrate predominates the Acetest may by negative. If there is concomitant lactic acidosis the anion gap will be excessively large for the degree of positivity of the nitroprusside reaction.
   c. *Starvation* frequently results in a mild ketoacidosis due to excessive fatty acid metabolism.
   d. *Alcoholic ketoacidosis* usually follows prolonged vomiting in association with excessive alcohol consumption. Since β hydroxybutyrate is the main anion produced in this setting the nitroprusside reaction may be negative.
   e. *Intoxication* with a variety of drugs and poisons may lead to overproduction of anions and an anion gap type metabolic acidosis. This is the typical acid-base disturbance that is seen in poisoning with salicylates, methanol (formate), ethylene glycol (oxalate) and paraldehyde

(acetoacetate).* *Note*: Salicylates may also cause respiratory alkalosis by direct stimulation of respiration (see below).

2. *Reduced elimination of acid*. The second major cause of increased anion-gap type metabolic acidosis is failure to eliminate endogenous or exogenous acid. This is the pathogenesis of the metabolic acidosis encountered in acute and chronic renal failure.

Management of metabolic acidosis
There are two main elements in the management of any acid-base disorder. Firstly the underlying disease process must be identified and treated. Secondly, if the acid-base disorder, e.g. severe lactic acidosis, is itself life threatening then immediate 'first-aid' measures aimed at restoring blood pH towards normal are required. In order to analyse a given acid-base disturbance it is first necessary to assess the adequacy or otherwise of physiological compensation. This process allows rapid analysis of mixed acid-base disorders.

In metabolic acidosis the primary disturbance is a reduction in plasma bicarbonate for any of the reasons outlined above. Respiratory compensation results in an increase in ventilation and hence a reduction in Pa_{CO_2}. When fully developed the magnitude of this compensatory response is related to the fall in plasma bicarbonate. As a rough rule of thumb Pa_{CO_2} should fall by around 1 kPa for every 7.5 mmol/l decrease in plasma bicarbonate.

A simple metabolic acidosis associated with a plasma bicarbonate over 15 mmol/l is best managed by treatment of the underlying disease since it is unlikely to result in a life-threatening blood pH. When plasma bicarbonate is less than 10 mmol/l bicarbonate therapy is usually required. The amount of bicarbonate required varies depending on the cause and severity of the acidosis. Patients with an increased anion-gap type metabolic acidosis have potential bicarbonate in forms such as lactate or acetoacetate. Assuming the underlying disease is satisfactorily treated such patients will ultimately require less exogenous base than a patient with the same degree of acidosis resulting from bicarbonate loss.

Over rapid correction of blood pH may lead to tetany or convulsions. It is thus recommended that only half of the estimated bicarbonate deficit be replaced in the first 12 hours. The amount of bicarbonate that should be given can be calculated for an apparent volume of distribution of bicarbonate

---

* The compounds in brackets are the principal unmeasured anions.

of 50% body weight. For example a 70 kg man has a plasma bicarbonate of 10 mmol/l. To increase the plasma bicarbonate to 17 mmol/l the patient needs $70 \times 0.5 \times 7 = 245$ mmol bicarbonate. This is a fairly typical bicarbonate deficit which serves to illustrate why giving bolus injections of 50 mmol bicarbonate has little or no impact on blood pH in severe metabolic acidosis.

Bicarbonate therapy is not without considerable risk, mainly volume overload and hypernatraemia from the large volumes of hypertonic sodium bicarbonate required to correct the acidosis. Hypokalaemia may also occur due to shifts of potassium into cells. This is especially likely in patients with diabetes or diarrhoea who tend to have substantial total body potassium deficits. Post-treatment alkalosis may result from giving too much alkali, from metabolism of, for example, lactate to produce endogenous bicarbonate, or from respiratory stimulation caused by persistent acidosis within the CSF.

Respiratory alkalosis
Respiratory alkalosis results from any stimulus (other than acidosis) which increases alveolar ventilation and hence reduces Pa_{CO_2}. Renal compensation for the reduced Pa_{CO_2} results in renal bicarbonate loss and a fall in plasma bicarbonate (Table 5). Since renal compensation is slow, requiring several days to become fully developed, the magnitude of the fall in plasma bicarbonate is smaller in acute respiratory alkalosis than in chronic respiratory alkalosis. As a general rule of thumb a fall in plasma bicarbonate of 2 mmol/l for every 1.3 kPa fall in Pa_{CO_2} is expected in acute respiratory alkalosis.

The causes of respiratory alkalosis are:

1. Central nervous system
   a. anxiety
   b. cerebrovascular accident
   c. trauma
   d. brain tumour
   e. meningitis/encephalitis
2. Respiratory
   a. pulmonary embolus
   b. pneumonia
   c. V/Q imbalance with hypoxia
   d. early pulmonary oedema
3. Other
   a. fever
   b. gram-negative septicaemia
   c. liver failure
   d. salicylates
   e. pregnancy

Table 5 Bicarbonate, pH and P_{CO_2} in simple acid-base disorders

	Plasma HCO_3	Plasma pH	Plasma P_{CO_2}
Metabolic acidosis	↓	↓	↓
alkalosis	↑	↑	↑
Respiratory acidosis	↑	↓	↑
alkalosis	↓	↑	↑

Chronic respiratory alkalosis is rather rare since most of the conditions which lead to respiratory alkalosis (see above) are short-lived. As a rough rule of thumb in chronic respiratory alkalosis plasma bicarbonate falls by 5 mmol/l for every 1.3 kPa fall in Pa_{CO_2}.

ELEVATED PLASMA BICARBONATE

This is characteristic of both metabolic alkalosis and respiratory acidosis. These conditions can usually be differentiated on the basis of the different clinical settings in which they occur. Where doubt remains they may be distinguished on the basis of blood pH which tends to be alkalaemic in metabolic alkalosis and acidaemic in respiratory acidosis.

Metabolic alkalosis
Metabolic alkalosis results from any condition which tends to elevate total plasma CO_2 and hence plasma bicarbonate. From a diagnostic and therapeutic standpoint it is convenient to subdivide metabolic alkalosis into chloride sensitive and chloride resistant. The major causes of metabolic alkalosis are:

1. Chloride responsive
    a. Vomiting
    b. Gastric suction
    c. Diuretics
        (i) thiazides
        (ii) loop diuretics
        (iii) metolazone
    d. Relief of chronic hypercapnia
2. Chloride resistant
    a. Hyperaldosteronism
        (i) primary
        (ii) secondary
    b. Cushing's syndrome
        (i) iatrogenic
        (ii) ectopic ACTH
        (iii) basophil adenoma
        (iv) adrenal

c. Bartter's syndrome
d. Liddle's syndrome
e. 11β and 17α hydroxylase deficiencies
f. Liquorice
g. Carbenoxolone
h. Severe potassium depletion

Chloride sensitive metabolic alkalosis
This occurs in situations where chloride is lost in excess of
sodium, e.g. in vomiting or gastric suction where chloride is lost
with hydrogen ion. The concomitant volume depletion results in
avid renal sodium conservation. Since no chloride is available to
be reabsorbed with sodium the kidney reabsorbs sodium
bicarbonate thus perpetuating the alkalosis. The most important
diagnostic test is urine chloride which will be very low or absent
in metabolic alkalosis of this type. Urine sodium is also low
except when e.g. continued vomiting means that bicarbonate
generation in continuing. In this situation excess bicarbonate is
lost via the kidneys along with sodium. In patients with
metabolic alkalosis due to diuretic loss the urine may, of course,
contain chloride if diuretic use is continuing, despite obvious
chloride depletion. Post-hypercapnic alkalosis results from the
selective renal chloride loss that is an adaptive response to
chronic hypercapnia. When the hypercapnia is abruptly relieved
the excess bicarbonate is retained by the kidney because there is
little available chloride with which to reabsorb sodium.

Chloride resistant metabolic alkalosis
This occurs in conditions where there is direct stimulation of
renal bicarbonate reabsorption, usually as the result of excessive
mineralocorticoid activity.
   Primary hyperaldosteronism presents as a hypokalaemic
metabolic alkalosis associated with hypertension and a plasma
sodium in the upper part of the normal range. Secondary
hyperaldosteronism also presents as hypokalaemic metabolic
alkalosis accompanied by features of the underlying disease, e.g.
nephrotic syndrome, cardiac failure. Cushing's syndrome,
including the iatrogenic and ectopic ACTH varieties, is an
important cause of metabolic alkalosis.
   Bartter's syndrome is characterised by hypokalaemic metabolic
alkalosis and normotension. Plasma aldosterone and renin are
both high and hyperplasia of the renal juxtaglomerular apparatus
is noted histologically. These patients are often volume depleted
at presentation and may be confused with those patients who
have surreptitious vomiting as a cause of alkalosis. The
distinction is made by urine chloride which is absent in
surreptitious vomiting and present in Barrter's syndrome.

Liddles's syndrome is very rare and presents similarly to primary hyperaldosteronism though plasma aldosterone is low. It is thought to be due to an as yet unidentified mineralocorticoid. Deficiency of adrenal 11β or 17α hydroxylases results in excessive production of desoxycorticosterone which has mineralocorticoid effects. Liquorice contains a mineralocorticoid (glycyrrhizinic acid) of which carbenoxolone is a derivative. Both may cause hypokalaemic metabolic alkalosis.

The role of uncomplicated hypokalaemia in causing metabolic alkalosis remains unclear. It is likely that profound hypokalaemia (plasma potassium < 2 mmol/l), associated with total body potassium deficits in excess of 500 mmol may lead directly to metabolic alkalosis, probably by direct effects on increasing renal ammonium and net acid excretion.

Management of metabolic alkalosis
Unlike metabolic acidosis, simple metabolic alkalosis is not a life-threatening acid-base disturbance. Therapy is thus directed at the underlying cause. In exceptional circumstances a rapid fall in plasma bicarbonate can be achieved by giving hydrogen ion as either oral ammonium chloride or intravenous arginine hydrochloride.

The adequacy of renal compensation for metabolic alkalosis should be assessed in order to detect mixed acid-base disorders. The normal respiratory response to an increase in plasma bicarbonate is hypoventilation. The degree of hypoventilation that occurs is limited because of the need for adequate oxygenation. It is thus rare to see Pa_{CO_2} rise above 6.6 kPa in uncomplicated metabolic alkalosis. As a rough rule of thumb Pa_{CO_2} should rise by no more than 1 kPa for every 10 mmol/l rise in plasma bicarbonate in simple metabolic alkalosis. The actual rise in Pa_{CO_2} may be considerably less than this.

Respiratory acidosis
Respiratory acidosis is the result of conditions (other than metabolic alkalosis) which result in a primary reduction in alveolar ventilation. The main causes are listed in Table 6. The clinical setting gives the clue to diagnosis in the majority of cases. The mechanism whereby hypercapnia is produced is usually obvious. More subtle perhaps is neuromuscular blockade produced or potentiated by aminoglycosides, particularly in patients with renal failure undergoing surgery with muscle relaxants.

Management of respiratory acidosis
Respiratory acidosis is best managed by appropriate therapy of the underlying cause. Many of the conditions listed in Table 6

Table 6 Causes of respiratory acidosis

	Acute	Chronic
CNS	sedative overdose general anaesthesia trauma CVA	primary alveolar hypoventilation Pickwickian syndrome tumour chronic sedation overdose
Respiratory	aspiration laryngospasm bronchospasm pneumothorax flail chest severe pneumonia	COAD kyphoscoliosis ankylosing spondylitis fibrosing alveolitis severe pneumonia
Neuromuscular	Guillain- Barre tetanus/botulism myasthenic crisis drugs (e.g. curare, aminoglycosides)	poliomyelitis multiple sclerosis amyotrophic lateral sclerosis myopathy
Other	cardiac arrest severe pulmonary oedema	myxoedema

cause abrupt, short-lived rises in Pa_{co_2}. Since renal adaptation is slow a sharp rise in Pa_{co_2} can cause a large rise in hydrogen ion concentration due to acute lack of buffer. Typically in acute respiratory acidosis plasma bicarbonate rises by only 2–3 mmol/l irrespective of the rise in Pa_{co_2}. Hydrogen ion concentration rises sharply in acute respiratory acidosis, the rise averaging 6 mmol/l for every 1 kPa increase in Pa_{co_2}. Thus if Pa_{co_2} rises from 5.28 to 7.28 kPa hydrogen ion concentration rises by 12 mmol/l, equivalent to a fall in pH to 7.28.

In chronic respiratory acidosis the renal adaptation is more complete. In this situation a 1 kPa rise in Pa_{co_2} will on average be accompanied by a rise in plasma bicarbonate of around 3 mmol/l.

Normal divalent ion metabolism

CALCIUM

Calcium plays a vital role in the regulation of neuromuscular function, myocardial contractility, hormone release and enzyme activity so that its intracellular and extracellular concentrations are closely controlled. Intracellular calcium concentration is controlled by mitochondrial and cell membrane transport while extracellular calcium concentrations depends on parathyroid hormone (PTH) and vitamin D.

In blood, calcium exists in three forms: (1) around 40% of calcium is bound to protein, mainly albumin; (2) about 15% of calcium is diffusible but complexed with phosphate, citrate and sulphate; and (3) the remaining 45% of serum calcium is free ionized calcium. It is the free ionized calcium that is biologically active. Total and ionized serum calcium may vary considerably depending on serum protein concentration and acid-base status. Thus increasing serum albumin (e.g. by venous stasis) will increase total serum calcium, ionized calcium being unchanged. Conversely, hypoalbuminaemia results in a fall in total calcium concentration. Systemic acidosis increases the proportion of serum calcium that is ionized by reducing protein binding. Alkalosis reduces serum ionized calcium by increasing protein binding.

Since ionized calcium is physiologically active it is necessary to estimate ionized calcium in certain clinical situations unless it can be measured directly. Such an estimate takes into account changes in ionized or total calcium induced by changes in pH or protein content of serum. At normal serum albumin, ionized calcium concentration varies by about 0.05 mmol/l for every 0.1 change in pH. At a constant pH, total calcium falls by around 0.025 mmol/l for every 1 g/l drop in serum albumin concentration from 40 g/l.

Calcium balance

Under normal physiological circumstances there is a strict balance between calcium intake and calcium excretion which can be varied according to calcium needs.

Calcium absorption
In a normal calcium replete individual up to a third of dietary
calcium is absorbed. Calcium absorption takes place largely in
the jejunum where it may be active and under control of vitamin
D (80–90%) or passive (10–20%). Active calcium absorption is in
part dependent on a calcium sensitive magnesium-dependent
ATP-ase so that magnesium deficiency may impair calcium
absorption.

On a normal dietary intake of 23 mmol (900 mg) calcium net
calcium absorption is around 7.5 mmol. In vitamin D deficient
states 'normal' calcium absorption can be achieved by passive
absorption if dietary calcium is increased to 75–100 mmol
(3–4 g). Calcium absorption shows adaptation to dietary calcium
in that vitamin D dependent calcium absorption can be increased
or decreased in response to low or high dietary calcium contents
respectively.

Calcium excretion
There are two principal routes of calcium excretion. A fixed
amount (3–4 mmol) is excreted in the distal small bowel and
large bowel. This calcium loss is obligatory and occurs even in
states of calcium deficiency. Renal calcium excretion is variable
and under the control of PTH. Urinary calcium excretion accounts
for final calcium balance, the amount appearing in urine being
adjusted to reflect net intestinal calcium absorption.

Renal handling of calcium is summarised in Figure 19. Briefly,
around 60% of total serum calcium (i.e. ionized and diffusible) is
filtered at the glomerulus giving a normal filtered load of around
270 mmol/24 hours. Around 60–65% of this is reabsorbed
passively in the proximal convoluted tubule along with sodium.
There is some evidence that calcium reabsorption in later
sections of the proximal convoluted tubule (the pars recta) is
active and can proceed against an electrochemical gradient.

Little or no calcium transport occurs in the thin descending or
ascending limbs of the loop of Henle. In the thick ascending loop
of Henle 20–25% of filtered calcium is passively reabsorbed in
parallel with sodium. In the distal convoluted tubule around 10%
of filtered calcium is reabsorbed by an active process that is PTH
sensitive and independent of sodium transport. Distal tubular
function determines final adjustment of urinary calcium excretion
which is less than 7.5 mmol/24 hours in adults and 0.1 mmol/kg
body weight in children.

Regulation of serum calcium
Calcium homeostasis is maintained by the balance between net
calcium absorption and urinary calcium excretion. There is a
constant flux of calcium between blood and bone fluid. However,

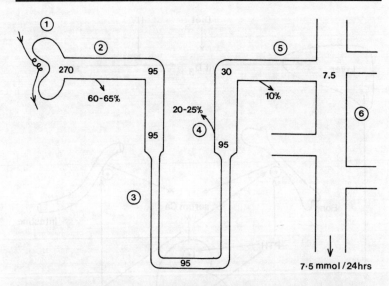

Fig. 19 Renal handling of calcium. Figures given are total amount of calcium (mmol/l). Percentages refer to percent of total filtered load reabsorbed in each segment of the nephron. 1. Glomerulus; 2. Proximal tubule; 3. Thin descending loop of Henle; 4. Thick ascending loop of Henle; 5. Distal tubule; 6. Collecting duct.

since bone formation and resorption normally proceed at the same rate there is no net loss or gain of calcium from bone. Serum calcium is therefore maintained by the balance of vitamin D dependent calcium absorption and PTH mediated release of calcium from bone and urinary calcium excretion (Fig. 20).

PHOSPHATE

Normal serum inorganic phosphate is 0.8–1.4 mmol/l. Intracellular phosphate (organic and inorganic) concentration is normally around 80 mmol/l. Total body phosphorus is normally around 20 000 mmol (~630 g) of which around 0.1% is in the extracellular fluid. About 85% of total body phosphorus is in bone but only about 0.6% of this (~100 mmol) is exchangeable with extracellular fluid.

Intracellular phosphorus is present in a wide range of organic phosphates, phospholipids and nucleotides which are vital to normal cell function. Inorganic phosphate is a major source of phosphorus for the synthesis of ATP and is thus of key importance in oxidative metabolism.

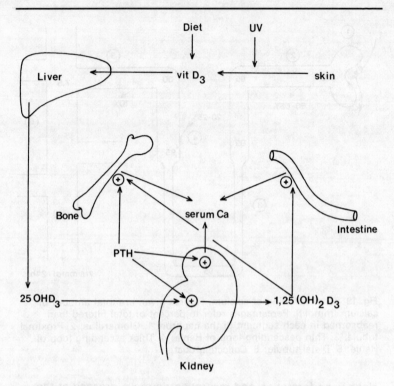

Fig. 20 Regulation of serum Ca. Serum Ca depends on interplay between bone resorption, calcium absorption and renal calcium excretion. + refers to stimulation by the appropriate hormone.

Intestinal phosphate transport

Phosphate is ingested in organic and inorganic forms. Most organic phosphate is hydrolyzed to and absorbed as inorganic phosphate in the gut, though some phospholipids are absorbed intact. In normal individuals a constant 60–65% of phosphate is absorbed over a wide range of dietary intakes.

Phosphate absorption takes place throughout the small intestine by either an active, vitamin D dependent mechanism that is distinct from that controlling calcium absorption, or by passive paracellular diffusion. The latter process accounts for the bulk of phosphate absorption.

Faecal phosphate is derived from unabsorbed dietary phosphate plus contributions from saliva, gastric, intestinal and pancreatic secretions and enterocyte turnover. Faecal phosphate ranges up to 20 mmol/24 hours depending on dietary intake.

Renal phosphate handling

Renal phosphate handling is summarised in Figure 21. There is a renal threshold for phosphate reabsorption (designated TmP/GFR) below which all filtered phosphate is reabsorbed and above which the excess filtered phosphate spills into the urine. The level of this reabsorptive threshold is largely dependent on PTH (see below). An increase in PTH results in a reduction in TmP/GFR with the result that more phosphate spills into the urine. The mechanism whereby the kidney reclaims phosphate is active transport at the sites indicated in Figure 21 mediated via a PTH sensitive adenylate cyclase.

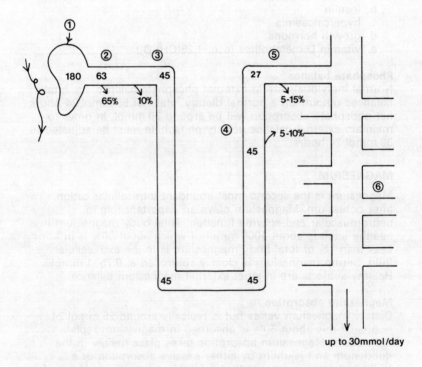

up to 30mmol/day

Fig. 21 Renal handling of phosphate. 1. Phosphate is freely filtered giving a daily filtered load of around 180 mmol. 2. Around 65% of phosphate is absorbed in the early proximal tubule and further 10% (3) in the pars recta. 4. 5–10% of filtered phosphate is absorbed in the thick segment of ascending loop of Henle. 5. Final adjustment of urinary phosphate occurs in the distal tubule with 5–15% of filtered phosphate being reabsorbed. Final urine phosphate depends on dietary intake. Phosphate reabsorption is at all points controlled by a PTH sensitive adenlyate cyclase.

Factors affecting renal phosphate reabsorption
1. Decrease phosphate reabsorption
   a. PTH
   b. high dietary PO_4
   c. ECF volume expansion
   d. diuretics
   e. calcitonin
   f. glucocorticoids
   g. thyroxine
   h. alcoholism
   i. alkaline urine
2. Increase phosphate reabsorption
   a. low dietary phosphate
   b. insulin
   c. hypercalcaemia
   d. growth hormone
   e. vitamin D metabolites (esp. $1,25(OH)_2D_3$)

Phosphate balance
Normal individuals are in external phosphate balance, i.e. intake balances output. On a normal dietary intake of 50 mmol/24 hours net phosphate absorption will be around 30 mmol. In order to maintain external balance urinary phosphate must be adjusted to 30 mmol/24 hours.

MAGNESIUM
Magnesium is the second most abundant intracellular cation, after potassium. Magnesium plays an important role in neuromuscular and enzyme function. Total body magnesium in a healthy adult is about 1000 mmol of which about 50% is in bone. Less than 1% of total body magnesium is in the extracellular fluid. Serum magnesium is closely controlled at 0.75–1 mmol/l. Healthy subjects are in strict external magnesium balance.

Magnesium absorption
Dietary magnesium varies but is typically around 25 mmol/24 hours. Of this about 50% is absorbed in magnesium replete individuals. Magnesium absorption takes place mainly in the duodenum and jejunum by either passive absorption or a facilitated passive process that is inhibited by calcium. A role for vitamin D in promoting magnesium absorption has not been conclusively shown.

A large number of factors influence intestinal magnesium absorption. It is enhanced by lactose, magnesium deficiency, low phosphate diet and high intraluminal sodium. Magnesium absorption is reduced by phytic acid, high dietary phosphate and high dietary calcium. Magnesium absorption is also increased by growth hormone, PTH and thyroxine and reduced by calcitonin and aldosterone.

Renal handling of magnesium

Renal handling of magnesium is markedly different from that of sodium or calcium (Fig. 22). Briefly, 75% of serum magnesium is ultrafiltrable giving a normal filtered load of around 120 mmol/24 hours. In the proximal tubule 15–30% of magnesium is reabsorbed passively (c.f. calcium and sodium). In the ascending loop of Henle 50–60% of filtered magnesium is passively reabsorbed. The ascending loop of Henle is thus the major site for both bulk reclamation of magnesium and adjustment of final urinary magnesium. Small but significant amounts of magnesium are passively reabsorbed at distal sites. Final urinary magnesium is variable and depends on net magnesium absorption and magnesium status. It is normally up to 20 mmol/24 hours.

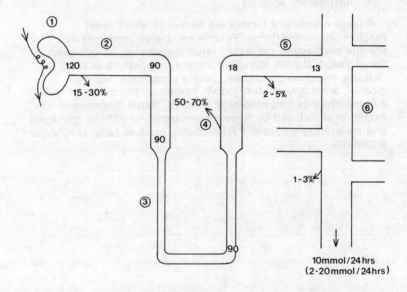

Fig. 22 Renal handling of magnesium. Figures given are total amount of magnesium (mmol/l). Percentages refer to percent of total filtered load reabsorbed at each segment of the nephron. 1. Glomerulus; 2. Proximal tubule; 3. Thin descending loop of Henle; 4. Thick ascending loop of Henle; 5. Distal tubule; 6. Collecting duct.

Factors regulating renal Mg excretion

1. Increase Mg excretion
   a. Volume contraction
   b. Renal vasodilatation
   c. Diuresis/natriuresis
   d. Hypermagnesaemia
   e. Dietary phosphate depletion
   f. Alcohol
   g. Aminoglycosides
   h. Growth hormone
   i. Thyroxine
   j. Adrenal steroids
   k. Metabolic acidosis
   e. Glucose/insulin
2. Reduce Mg excretion
   a. Volume expansion
   b. Hypomagnesaemia
   c. Calcitonin
   d. Glucagon
   e. Metabolic alkalosis
   f. Respiratory acidosis

A large number of factors are known to affect renal magnesium reabsorption. Volume expansion increases and volume contraction decreases renal magnesium reabsorption. Renal vasodilatation increases urinary magnesium as does diuresis, hypermagnesaemia, dietary phosphate depletion, alcohol, aminoglycosides, growth hormone, thyroxine, glucose, adrenal steroids and metabolic acidosis. Renal magnesium excretion is reduced by hypomagnesaemia, calcitonin, glucagon and respiratory acidosis. PTH probably reduces renal magnesium excretion.

Disorders of divalent ion metabolism

CALCIUM

At the clinical level disorders of calcium metabolism are manifested as hypo-or hypercalcaemia accompanied by features of the causative disorder.

HYPERCALCAEMIA

The main causes of hypercalcaemia are:
1. Tumours
   a. metastatic bone resorption
   b. ectopic PTH
   c. osteolysis
      (i) osteoclast activity factor
      (ii) osteolytic sterols
      (iii) prostaglandins
2. Primary hyperparathyroidism
   a. adenoma
   b. hyperplasia (incl. multiple endocrine neoplasia and familial)
3. Endocrine
   a. thyrotoxicosis
   b. acromegaly
   c. phaeochromocytoma
   d. glucocorticoid deficiency
4. Granulomatous disorders
   a. sarcoidosis
   b. tuberculosis
   c. berylliosis
   d. histoplasmosis
   e. coccidiomycosis
5. Thiazide diuretics
6. Immobilization
7. Paget's disease
8. Milk-alkali syndrome
9. Hypervitaminosis D and A

10. Post-renal transplant
11. Recovery phase of ATN
12. Lithium
13. Familial hypocalciuric hypercalcaemia

Symptomatic hypercalcaemia is rare while asymptomatic
hypercalcaemia may be found in up to 0.1% of the population, in
association with a wide variety of disorders. Malignancy and
hyperparathyroidism together account for around 75% of all
cases of hypercalcaemia

Tumour related hypercalcaemia
This may result from bone resorption due to metastatic invasion
(e.g. carcinoma of prostate), from eleboration of a PTH like
substance by the tumour (e.g. carcinoma of breast or bronchus)
or from the release of osteolytic factors. The latter include
osteoclast activating factor (OAF), osteolytic vitamin D like sterols
and prostaglandins.

Primary hyperparathyroidism
This causes hypercalcaemia through a PTH mediated increase in
calcium release from bone and an indirect increase in intestinal
calcium absorption mediated by PTH stimulation of renal
$1,25(OH)_2D_3$ synthesis. Around 80% of patients with primary
hyperparathyroidism have a single adenoma and 15% have
diffuse hyperplasia. A small proportion have multiple
adenomatas while up to 3% have functional parathyroid
carcinomas.

Endocrine disorders
A variety of endocrine disorders may give rise to hypercalcaemia.
In *thyrotoxicosis* 10–20% of patients are hypercalcaemic although
ionized calcium is elevated in up to 40%. The aetiology is
thyroxine mediated bone resorption. In *acromegaly* 15–20% of
patients are hypercalcaemic. The cause is unknown but may be
increased production of $1,25(OH)_2D_3$ with subsequent increase in
intestinal calcium absorption and bone resorption. In
phaeochromocytoma hypercalcaemia is rare. It is thought to
result from direct effect of catecholamines on bone resorption or
stimulation of PTH release by catecholamines. In *hypoadrenalism*
significant hypercalcaemia is rare. The exact cause is unknown
though it is suggested that intestinal calcium absorption may be
enhanced in the absence of glucocorticoids.

Granulomatous disorders
These are uncommon causes of hypercalcaemia. In *sarcoidosis*
the reported incidence of hypercalcaemia varies from 1 to 20%.

The cause is increased production of $1,25(OH)_2D_3$ which, in sarcoidosis, seems to take place within the sarcoid granulomas, i.e. it is extra-renal. The incidence of hypercalcaemia in other granulomatous disorders is low but the aetiology is probably the same.

Thiazide diuretics
These frequently cause hypercalcaemia, particularly in patients with underlying bone disease such as hyperparathyroidism or multiple myeloma. The aetiology is multifactorial with haemoconcentration, reduced urinary calcium excretion and enhanced bone resorption all contributing to the hypercalcaemia.

Immobilization
This usually results in hypercalciuria though occasionally hypercalcaemia may occur. During immobilization bone resorption occurs more quickly than bone formation. Any situation in which bone turnover rate is already increased, e.g. Paget's disease, young children or teenagers, is therefore associated with an increased incidence of hypercalcaemia during immobilization.

Paget's disease
This disease of the bone rarely causes hypercalcaemia except during periods of immobilization.

Milk-alkali syndrome
This syndrome is now very rare. The oral ingestion of 5–10 g of calcium along with absorbable alkali (e.g. sodium bicarbonate) causes hypercalcaemia, nephrocalcinosis and ultimately renal failure. The systemic alkalosis that accompanies alkali ingestion lowers urine calcium excretion. Intestinal calcium absorption is increased by the non-vitamin D dependent route, even if vitamin D dependent absorption is completely inhibited.

Hypervitaminosis D
This usually complicates treatment of hypoparathyroidism with vitamin D but may rarely be seen in patients deliberately ingesting large amounts of vitamin D. It is due to vitamin D mediated increases in intestinal calcium absorption and bone resorption. *Hypervitaminosis A* is a rare cause of hypercalcaemia seen most frequently in haemodialysis patients. The hypercalcaemia is due to enhanced osteoclastic bone resorption.

Post-renal transplant
Hypercalcaemia can occur in up to a third of patients receiving successful renal transplants. It is usually mild and transient and results from persistent hyperparathyroidism.

Recovery phase of acute tubular necrosis
The recovery phase of ATN is complicated by hypercalcaemia in up to 25% of those cases due to a non-traumatic rhabdomyolysis. The hypercalcaemia is due to persistence of secondary hyperparathyroidism induced by hypocalcaemia during the oliguric phase of ATN. Dissolution of soft tissue calcifications in damaged muscle may also contribute to the hypercalcaemia.

Lithium
This is a rare cause of hypercalcaemia, probably mediated by increased PTH secretion.

Familial hypocalciuric hypercalcaemia
This is an autosomal dominant disorder characterized by hypercalcaemia, mild hypermagnesaemia, normal renal function and a reduced fractional urinary calcium excretion. Tubular calcium reabsorption is increased suggesting an increased sensitivity of renal tubules to PTH or cAMP as the underlying mechanism.

Clinical features of hypercalcaemia
1. Non-specific—features of underlying condition
2. Cardiovascular
   a. ECG—short QT interval
   b. hypertension
   c. potentiates digoxin toxicity
3. Gastrointestinal
   a. anorexia, nausea, vomiting
   b. peptic ulcer
   c. constipation
   d. pancreatitis
4. Renal
   a. polyuria, nocturia, polydipsia
   b. acute/chronic renal failure
   c. nephrolithiasis/nephrocalcinosis
5. Metastatic calcification
6. Neurological—confusion, stupor, coma

Approach to the patient with hypercalcaemia
An approach to the diagnosis of hypercalcaemia is given in Figure 23.

Non-specific features of the underlying disease
These include, for example, anorexia and weight loss in malignancy, myopathy and bone pain in hyperparathyroidism or rash and lymphadenopathy in sarcoidosis. A careful history and physical examination will provide clues to the presence of one of

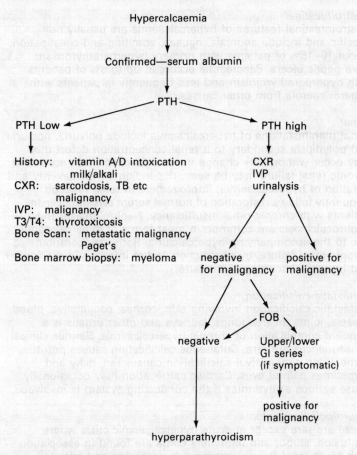

Fig. 23 Approach to the patient with hypercalcaemia.

the major causes of hypercalcaemia which can then be confirmed by appropriate laboratory tests.

Cardiovascular
Cardiovascular problems are common in hypercalcaemia. The most characteristic change on ECG is shortening of the QT interval. Since hypercalcaemia increases cardiac contractility, toxicity of digoxin is potentiated while severe hypercalcaemia per se may precipitate ventricular tachycardia or ventricular fibrillation. Up to 30% of patients with hyperparathyroidism have hypertension which is improved by removal of the adenoma in about half.

Gastrointestinal
Gastrointestinal features of hypercalcaemia are usually non-specific and include anorexia, nausea, vomiting and constipation. About 10–15% of patients with primary hyperparathyroidism have peptic ulcers. Pancreatitis occurs in up to 8% of patients with hyperparathyroidism and less frequently in patients with hypercalcaemia from other causes.

Renal
Renal manifestations of hypercalcaemia include polyuria, nocturia and polydipsia secondary to a renal concentration defect that may occur without any change in renal function. Both acute and chronic renal failure may be seen, depending on the severity and duration of hypercalcaemia. Improvement in renal function frequently follows restoration of normal serum calcium even in patients with chronic renal insufficiency. Nephrolithiasis and nephrocalcinosis are common in most forms of hypercalcaemia due to the accompanying hypercalciuria. Both may contribute to chronic renal failure, by obstruction and/or infection in the former and interstitial scarring in the latter.

Metastatic calcification
Metastatic calcification involving skin, cornea, conjunctiva, blood vessels, joints, hearts, lungs, kidneys and other organs is a frequent complication of chronic hypercalcaemia. Serious clinical consequences are rare. Cutaneous calcification causes pruritus, corneal and conjunctival calcification causes red, itchy and sometimes painful eyes. Cardiac calcification may occasionally cause serious arrhythmias if the conducting system is involved.

Neurological symptoms
These are rare except in acute hypercalcaemic crisis where confusion, stupor and ultimately coma are found in association with acute renal failure, vomiting, hypotension and muscle weakness. This syndrome is rare and is seen most frequently in primary hyperparathyroidism.

Treatment of hypercalcaemia
The major treatment modalities for hypercalcaemia are summarised in Table 7. Treatment of any individual patient with hypercalcaemia may utilise a combination of the therapies outlined in Table 7 that is determined by the clinical situation.

Acute symptomatic hypercalcaemia
This demands urgent treatment. The patient is usually volume depleted so that volume expansion should be the first treatment. If hypercalcaemia is mild to moderate volume expansion alone may be sufficient to control the hypercalcaemia. At serum

Table 7 Treatment of hypercalcaemia

Treatment	Indications	Method	Advantages	Disadvantages
Oral or I.V. phosphate	Mild to moderate hypercalcaemia	1.5–3 g elemental phosphate daily. I.V. phosphate not recommended	Rapid effect	Causes metastatic calcification esp. I.V.
Calcitonin	moderate to severe hypercalcaemia	4μ/kg I.V. then 4μ/kg s.c. 12–24 hrs later	Rapid effect	Ineffective in up to 25%. Resistance limits chronic use.
Mithramycin	moderate to severe hypercalcaemia	25 μg/kg I.V. repeated as necessary	Rapid effect	Repeated use may cause thrombocytopaenia, liver dysfunction
Steroids	sarcoid, myeloma some tumours, vitamin D intoxication	0.5–1 mg/kg prednisolone daily. 3–5 mg/kg hydrocortisone daily	Relatively non-toxic	Slow onset (2–3 days)
Saline diuresis	acute hypercalcaemia	Prime with 1–2 l saline I.V. frusemide 40–80 mg every 2–3 hrs. Replace K$^+$ and Mg^{2+} if diuresis prolonged	Very rapidly effective	Needs renal function. May worsen volume depletion. Risk of hypokalaemia and hypomagnesaemia
EDTA	acute hypercalcaemia	15–50 mg I.V. over 4 hrs.	Very rapid	Nephrotoxic at high doses
Dialysis	acute hypercalcaemia and renal failure	Use calcium free dialysate. Haemo- or peritoneal dialysis	Very rapid	Vascular access & other dialysis related complications

calciums in excess of 3.7 mmol/l acute neurological symptoms and renal failure are usually present and there is a substantial risk of cardiac dysrhythmias. In most cases saline diuresis plus calcitonin or mithramycin is adequate. Calcitonin and mithramycin are effective even in renal failure. If renal failure is severe, calcium free dialysis should be used in place of saline diuresis. Corticosteroids have no place in the management of hypercalcaemic crisis.

Chronic hypercalcaemia
Treatment of chronic hypercalcaemia depends on the cause. Corticosteroids may be effective in sarcoidosis, myeloma, up to 50% of breast malignancies, vitamin D intoxication and immobilization. Oral phosphate is the treatment of choice in hyperparathyroidism (pending surgery) and most other malignancies. Mithramycin is reserved for patients unresponsive to phosphate or who have an elevated serum phosphate.

HYPOCALCAEMIA

The major causes of hypocalcaemia are:
1. Hypoalbuminaemia
2. Parathyroid dysfunction
   a. Hypoparathyroidism
       (i) surgical
      (ii) idiopathic
     (iii) infiltrative
   b. Pseudohypoparathyroidism
   c. Pseudoidiopathic hypoparathyroidism
3. Hypomagnesaemia
4. Abnormal vitamin D metabolism
   a. nutritional vitamin D deficiency
   b. malabsorption
   c. liver disease—reduced 25-OH D_3 synthesis
   d. accelerated 25–OH D_3 metabolism–phenytoin, phenobarbitone, alcohol, glutethimide
   e. accelerated loss of 25-OH D_3—nephrotic syndrome
   f. decreased 1,25(OH)$_2D_3$ synthesis—renal failure, vitamin D dependent rickets
5. Removal of calcium from serum
   a. hyperphosphataemia
   b. osteoblastic metastases
   c. acute pancreatitis
   d. hungry bone syndrome

Hypoalbuminaemia
This reduces total serum calcium by reducing the fraction of protein bound calcium. Serum ionized calcium is normal and there are no symptoms of hypocalcaemia.

Parathyroid dysfunction

This causes hypocalcaemia as a result of lack of PTH mediated bone resorption and low calcium absorption due to reduced $1,25(OH)_2D_3$ production.

1. *Hypoparathyroidism* may result from accidental injury to or removal of the parathyroids during neck surgery, especially thyroidectomy, where the incidence is about 3%.
2. *Idiopathic hypoparathyroidism* is rare. It presents most commonly in childhood or adolescence. There is an early onset familial type with X-linked inheritance. Late onset familial types with variable inheritance may be associated with pernicious anaemia, adrenal insufficiency, moniliasis and hypothyroidism.
   In both idiopathic and surgical hypoparathyroidism PTH and $1,25(OH)_2D_3$ concentrations are low and hypocalcaemia is associated with hyperphosphataemia.
3. *Pseudohypoparathyroidism* is characterised by hypocalcaemia, hyperphosphataemia, obesity, round face and short digits. The exact mode of inheritace is uncertain but is probably X-linked. The aetiology of the hypocalcaemia in pseudohypoparathyroidism appears to be end- organ resistance to the effects of PTH which results in a lack of PTH mediated bone resorption and low circulating $1,25(OH)_2D_3$ concentrations, despite normal or high PTH levels.
4. *Pseudoidiopathic hypoparathyroidism*. These patients have hypocalcaemia, hyperphosphatemia and high or normal PTH concentrations but lack the skeletal abnormalities of pseudohypoparathyroidism. They respond normally to PTH infusion and are thought to secrete a PTH that is biologically inactive.

Hypomagnesaemia

This causes hypocalcaemia principally by reducing PTH secretion and impairing skeletal responsiveness to PTH. This is important in managing patients with both hypocalcaemia and hypomagnesaemia since successful treatment of the hypocalcaemia requires correction of the hypomagnesaemia.

Abnormal vitamin D metabolism

This causes hypocalcaemia by means of reduced $1,25(OH)_2D_3$ production and consequent calcium malabsorption.

1. *Nutritional vitamin D deficiency* reduces the amount of $25\text{-}OHD_3$ available for production of $1,25(OH)_2D_3$. Typically there is hypocalcaemia, hypophosphataemia, secondary hyperparathyroidism and elevated bone alkaline phosphatase. In children vitamin D deficiency causes rickets and in adults osteomalacia.

2. *Malabsorption* of fat soluble vitamins in, for example, coeliac disease or chronic pancreatitis, may cause vitamin D deficient rickets or osteomalacia.
3. *Chronic liver disease* may be associated with a vitamin D resistant rickets or osteomalacia due to reduced conversion of vitamin D to 25-OHD$_3$. This in turn reduces 1,25(OH)$_2$D$_3$ production.
4. *Accelerated loss of 25-OHD$_3$* occurs in nephrotic syndrome as a result of loss of 25-OHD$_3$ bound to albumin in the urine. Interference with enterohepatic circulation of 25-OHD$_3$, e.g. ileal resection, may also cause vitamin D deficiency.
5. *Decreased 1,25(OH)$_2$D$_3$ synthesis* occurs in renal failure as a result of reduced nephron mass. Vitamin D dependent rickets (VDDR) is a rare autosomal recessive disorder. Clinically it resembles nutritional vitamin D deficiency but requires high doses of vitamin D to effect an improvement. In contrast, physiological doses of 1,25(OH)$_2$D$_3$ produce dramatic improvement suggesting VDDR results from an inherited lack of renal 25-OHD$_3$ 1α hydroxylase. A further type of VDDR (Type II) has been described in which serum 1,25(OH)$_2$D$_3$ is high, suggesting end-organ unresponsiveness to 1,25(OH)$_2$D$_3$ as the aetiology.

Removal of calcium from serum
This is an infrequent cause of hypocalcaemia
1. *Hyperphosphataemia* causes hypocalcaemia by reducing bone resorption, by impairing conversion of 25-OHD$_3$ to 1,25(OH)$_2$D$_3$ and by causing extravascular calcification. The main causes of hyperphosphataemia are listed on p. 85.
2. *Osteoblastic metastatic cancer* causes hypocalcaemia by removing calcium from the blood for new bone formation.
3. In *acute pancreatitis* hypocalcaemia occurs secondary to formation of calcium soaps in the pancreatic bed and to widespread calcification in subcutaneous fat. The degree of hypocalcaemia correlates with the severity of pancreatitis.
4. The *hungry bone syndrome* refers to situations where bone formation exceeds resorption and calcium is deposited in previously unmineralized bone with subsequent hypocalcaemia. Examples include successful surgical management of primary or secondary hyperparathyroidism and thyrotoxicosis or during treatment of nutritional vitamin D deficiency.

Clinical features of hypocalcaemia
The major symptoms and signs of hypocalcaemia are:
1. Neuromuscular
     tetany, paraesthesia, myopathy, seizures, extrapyramidal signs, Chvostek's sign, Trousseau's sign

2. Psychiatric
   impaired cognitive function, psychoses
3. Ophthalmological
   papilloedema, cataracts
4. Ectodermal/dental
   dry skin, nail dysplasia, moniliasis, defective tooth formation, defective enamel, root hypoplasia
5. Cardiovascular
   hypotension, reduced myocardial function, ECG—prolonged QT interval
6. Skeletal
   depends on underlying disease

Patients with hypocalcaemia usually have symptoms and signs of their underlying disease in addition to tetany, paraesthesiae or muscle spasms. An approach to the diagnosis of hypocalcaemia is given in Figure 24.

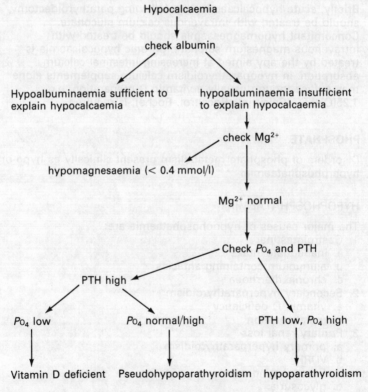

Fig. 24 Approach to the patient with hypocalcaemia.

Management of hypocalcaemia
1. Acute hypocalcaemia
     Ca gluconate 20–30 ml 10% over 10–15 mins. $MgSO_4$
     10–20 ml 10% 1.V. over 20–30 mins if hypomagnesaemic
     Treat as for chronic hypocalcaemia if hypocalcaemia persists
2. Chronic hypocalcaemia
   a. hypoparathyroidism
        calcium 2–4 g daily
        vitamin D 1.25–3.75 mg daily
        $1,25(OH)_2D_3$ 0.25–1μg daily
   b. vitamin D deficiency: depends on cause
        (i) nutritional—2–10 μg/24 hours vitamin D
        (ii) malabsorption—100–300 μg/24 hours vitamin D
        (iii) anticonvulsant—250 μg/24 hours vitamin D
        (iv) renal failure—0.25–1 μg $1,25(OH)_2D_3$ per 24 hours
        (v) VDDR Type I—0.25–1 μg $1,25(OH)_2D_3$ per 24 hours
        (vi) VDDR Type II—10–20 μg $1,25(OH)_2D_3$ per 24 hours

Briefly, acute hypocalcaemia, e.g. following parathyroidectomy,
should be treated with intravenous calcium gluconate.
Concomitant hypomagnesaemia should be treated with
intravenous magnesium sulphate. Chronic hypocalcaemia is
treated by therapy aimed at increasing intestinal calcium
absorption. In hypoparathyroidism calcium supplements alone
may suffice though usually a vitamin D preparation, e.g.
$1,25(OH)_2D_3$ (Calcitriol=Rocaltrol, Roche), is required.

PHOSPHATE

Disorders of phosphate metabolism present clinically as hypo-or
hyperphosphataemia.

HYPOPHOSPHATAEMIA

The major causes of hypophosphataemia are:
1. Gastrointestinal
   a. inadequate intake
   b. aluminium containing antacids
   c. chronic diarrhoea
2. Secondary hyperparathyroidism
   a. vitamin D deficiency
   b. malabsorption
3. Primary renal loss
   a. primary hyperparathyroidism
   b. VDRR
   c. Fanconi syndrome
   d. glycosuria
   e. diuretics

  f. volume expansion
  g. hypokalaemia
  h. hypomagnesaemia
4. Redistribution
  a. insulin/glucose administration
  b. hyperalimentation
  c. acute respiratory alkalosis
  d. catecholamines
5. Miscellaneous
  a. alcoholism
  b. diabetic ketoacidosis
  c. post-renal transplant

Gastrointestinal disturbances
These may cause mild to moderate hypophosphataemia.
Inadequate intake per se rarely causes hypophosphataemia but
makes its rapid development likely in the clinical situations listed
above. Chronic diarrhoea and aluminium containing antacids not
infrequently cause mild hypophosphataemia.

Secondary hyperparathyroidism
This can cause hypophosphataemia, for example in vitamin D
deficiency or malabsorption, by increasing renal phosphate
excretion. It is usually mild.

Primary renal loss
This loss of phosphate occurs in a number of conditions that on
occasion may cause severe hypophosphataemia. Vitamin D
resistant rickets (VDRR) is an X linked condition characterised by
hypophosphataemia and rickets unresponsive to physiological
doses of vitamin D. The primary abnormality is impaired
proximal phosphate reabsorption.
  The Fanconi syndrome results from proximal tubular damage
and links hypophosphataemia and phosphaturia with glucosuria,
uricosuria, aminoaciduria and bicarbonaturia. The main causes of
Fanconi syndrome are:

1. Inherited
  a. cystinosis
  b. galactosaemia
  c. Wilson's disease
  d. fructose intolerance
  e. Lowe's syndrome
  f. tyrosinaemia
  g. adult Fanconi syndrome
2. Acquired
  a. myeloma
  b. amyloidosis

   c. light chain disease
   d. Sjögren's syndrome
   e. renal transplantation
   f. primary hyperparathyroidism
   g. heavy metals—cadmium, mercury, lead
   h. drugs/toxins—salicylates, neomycin, outdated tetracycline,
       nitrobenzene, maleic acid

Diuretic therapy and volume expansion may both cause
phosphaturia and hence hypophosphataemia. Prolonged
hypokalaemia or hypomagnesaemia occasionally cause
phosphaturia and hypophosphataemia. Glycosuria causes renal
phosphate wasting because glucose competes with phosphate for
proximal reabsorption.

Redistribution
Redistribution of phosphate into cells is an important cause of
often severe hypophosphataemia. Administration of glucose and
insulin, e.g. during hyperalimentation, leads to
hypophosphataemia due to movement of phosphate into cells to
participate in intracellular metabolism. Acute respiratory alkalosis,
e.g. due to fever, sepsis or mechanical ventilation also causes
redistribution of phosphate into cells, as does the administration
of catecholamines.

Miscellaneous causes
Miscellaneous causes of hypophosphataemia include *alcoholism*
where the aetiology of hypophosphataemia is multifactorial. In
the hospitalized alcoholic the combination of a previously
inadequate diet, carbohydrate loading and respiratory alkalosis
(with the onset of delirium tremens) often produces profound
hypophosphataemia. Up to a third of patients with a successful
renal transplant develop transient hypophosphataemia due to a
combination of persistent hyperparathyroidism, primary tubular
phosphate leak and hungry bones. In *diabetic ketoacidosis*
hypophosphataemia occurs in part due to renal phosphate
wasting secondary to glycosuria and in part due to redistribution
of phosphate into cells during therapy. Severe
hypophosphataemia may occur during therapy of diabetic
ketoacidosis.

Symptoms and signs of hypophosphataemia
Symptomatic hypophosphataemia is rare and is seen most often
in diabetic ketoacidosis, alcoholics, during hyperalimentation and
following renal transplantation. Profound myopathy may occur
with elevation in serum creatine kinase and even frank
rhabdomyolysis. Cardiomyopathy may occur with prolonged
hypophosphataemia. Coma and seizures are rare.

Osteomalacia/rickets is seen with severe prolonged hypophosphataemia and may respond to phosphate repletion alone.

Treatment of hypophosphataemia

Initial treatment should be directed at the underlying disease. In mild to moderate hypophosphataemia this may be sufficient to treat the hypophosphataemia. Severe symptomatic hypophosphataemia always requires phosphate repletion. Phosphate supplements are usually given orally since I.V. replacement is complicated by risks of hyperphosphataemia or metastatic calcification. In general phosphate supplementation need not exceed 200 mmol/24 hours though therapy may need to be prolonged if phosphate depletion is severe. The exception to the rule on replacement of phosphate I.V. is during hyperalimentation where around 40 mmol of phosphate should be given for every 1000 kcal of energy supplied as carbohydrate.

HYPERPHOSPHATAEMIA

The principal causes of hyperphosphataemia are:
1. Increased phosphate load
   a. Endogenous
      (i) cytotoxic therapy
      (ii) rhabdomyolysis
   b. Exogenous
      (i) phosphate enemas
      (ii) laxative abuse
      (iii) I.V. phosphate therapy
      (iv) vitamin D intoxication
2. Reduced glomerular filtration rate
   acute or chronic renal failure
3. Increased tubular reabsorption
   a. hypoparathyroidism
   b. pseudohypoparathyroidism
   c. thyrotoxicosis
   d. acromegaly
   e. EHDP (diphosphonate)
   f. tumoural calcinosis

Increased phosphate load
A massive increase in the amount of phosphate presented to the kidneys may overwhelm their capacity to excrete it. Hyperphosphataemia may result.
1. Endogenous sources of a massive phosphate load include cytotoxic therapy, especially of lymphomas or leukaemias, and acute rhabdomyolysis from a variety of causes such as crush injury, seizures, electric shock, hyperthermia or drug

overdosage. Rhabdomyolysis is not infrequently associated with acute renal failure which further compromises renal phosphate excretion, worsening the hyperphosphataemia.
2. *Exogenous* sources of massive phosphate loading include phosphate enemas, particularly in patients with laxative abuse which results in increased colonic permeability to phosphate. Hyperphosphataemia due to intravenous phosphate is not uncommon during I.V. feeding or therapy of hypophosphataemia. Vitamin D intoxication increases intestinal phosphate absorption. Since TmP/GFR is high because PTH is suppressed by the accompanying hypercalcaemia, renal phosphate excretion is reduced, resulting in hyperphosphataemia.

Reduced glomerular filtration rate
Both acute and chronic renal failure result in hyperphosphataemia due to inability of the kidneys to excrete even a normal phosphate load. In chronic renal failure progressive secondary hyperparathyroidism, by increasing renal phosphate excretion, prevents severe hyperphosphataemia until GFR falls below 25–30 ml/min.

Increased tubular reabsorption
A variety of disorders cause hyperphosphataemia by increasing TmP/GFR.
1. *Hypoparathyroidism* from any cause produces hyperphosphataemia via the increase in tubular phosphate reabsorption that occurs when PTH is absent.
2. *Pseudohypoparathyroidism* also produces hyperphosphataemia by increasing TmP/GFR. However, PTH concentrations are high in this condition which results from a renal tubular insensitivity to circulating PTH. Pseudohyperhypoparathyroidism is a variant in which the renal tubules are insensitive to PTH but the bones respond normally. These patients have hyperphosphataemia and skeletal changes of hyperparathyroidism.
3. *Thyrotoxicosis* produces hyperphosphataemia partly by increasing TmP/GFR, partly by increasing intestinal phosphate absorption and phosphate release from bone.
4. *In acromegaly* a direct effect of growth hormone on increasing phosphate reabsorption may cause mild hyperphosphataemia.
5. *EHDP* (disodium ethane hydroxy diphosphonate) is used in the treatment of Paget's disease. It is a potent stimulator of renal phosphate reabsorption. Its use is usually accompanied by mild hyperphosphataemia.
6. *Tumoral calcinosis* is a familial disorder, commoner in negros, characterized by hyperphosphataemia and widespread soft-tissue calcifications. PTH concentrations and serum calcium

are normal. It is due to a primary increase in renal phosphate reabsorption.

Signs and symptoms of hyperphosphataemia
The signs and symptoms of hyperphosphataemia are those of hypocalcaemia and soft-tissue calcification. Acute hyperphosphataemia may present with tetany, hypotension, acute renal failure and arrhythmias due to cardiac calcification. Chronic hyperphosphataemia is associated with secondary hyperparathyroidism due to the coincident hypocalcaemia. Symptoms are therefore myopathy, osteitis fibrosa, soft-tissue calcification (pruritus, conjunctivitis, band keratopathy).

Treatment of hyperphosphataemia
Severe acute hyperphosphataemia may be life threatening. If renal function is normal, removal of the cause results in resolution of the hyperphosphataemia. Acetazolamide may be used to alkalinize the urine and enhance phosphate excretion. If renal function is impaired, haemodialysis may be required.

Chronic hyperphosphataemia is usually due to chronic renal failure. It is treated by dietary phosphate restriction and oral administration of phosphate binding antacids such as aluminium hydroxide or calcium carbonate. Chronic hyperphosphataemia also responds to haemodialysis though oral phosphate binders may still be required.

MAGNESIUM

Disorders of magnesium metabolism present clinically as hypo- or hypermagnesaemia

HYPERMAGNESAEMIA

The principal causes of hypermagnesaemia are:
1. Renal failure—acute or chronic
2. Reduced renal magnesium excretion with no change in GFR
    a. Salt depletion
    b. mineralocorticoid deficiency
    c. hypothyroidism
    d. chronic hypercapnia
3. Administration of magnesium
    a. antacids/laxative abuse
    b. magnesium therapy of seizures
    c. high magnesium dialysate
4. Tissue breakdown
    a. rhabdomyolysis
    b. burns
    c. diabetic ketoacidosis

Renal failure
This is commonly associated with hypermagnesaemia which may occasionally be severe. It is seen in both acute and chronic renal failure but is commoner and more severe in acute renal failure. In chronic renal failure it is a late phenomenon.
Hypermagnesaemia can be readily precipitated in patients with renal failure following the administration of magnesium containing antacids or laxatives. These should be avoided in patients with renal failure.

Reduced renal magnesium excretion
This may occur without any change in GFR. In *salt depletion* tubular magnesium reabsorption is increased and mild hypermagnesaemia may occur. *Mineralocorticoid deficiency* promotes renal magnesium reabsorption as does hypothyroidism and the respiratory acidosis associated with *chronic hypercapnia.*

Administration of pharmacological doses of magnesium
This rarely causes significant hypermagnesaemia except in patients with renal impairment. It is seen most frequently during administration of magnesium containing antacids, laxatives or enemas. Magnesium sulphate therapy of seizures, e.g. in eclampsia, may occasionally cause hypermagnesaemia. In haemodialysis patients hypermagnesaemia occurs if a high magnesium dialysate is inadvertently used.

Increased tissue breakdown
This can lead to hypermagnesaemia by releasing magnesium from cells. Examples are severe rhabdomyolysis, burns or diabetic ketoacidosis.

Clinical features and therapy of hypermagnesaemia
The clinical features of hypermagnesaemia are:
1. Depressed neuromuscular function
   a. Reduced/absent deep tendon reflexes (Mg > 3.1 mmol/l)
   b. Paralysis of voluntary muscle (Mg > 5 mmol/l)
   c. Stupor, coma (Mg > 6.3 mmol/l)
2. Cardiovascular
   a. Hypotension (Mg > 2 mmol/l)
   b. Increased PR, QRS, QT. Intraventricular conduction problems (Mg > 3.1 mmol/l)
   c. Complete heart block, asystole (Mg > 7.5 mmol/l)

Therapy is aimed first at removing the underlying cause of the hypermagnesaemia if possible and secondly at removal of excess magnesium. If symptomatic hypermagnesaemia is associated with renal failure dialysis may be indicated.

Symptomatic therapy of hypermagnesaemia includes assisted ventilation for severe respiratory depression and intravenous calcium which has a specific antagonistic effect on the cardiac effects of magnesium.

HYPOMAGNESAEMIA

The causes of hypomagnesaemia are given below. This list is intended to be comprehensive so that only a brief discussion of each group of causes will follow:

1. Reduced intake
   a. protein- calorie malnutrition
   b. starvation
   c. prolonged I.V. therapy
2. Reduced intestinal absorption
   a. malabsorption
   b. small bowel resection
   c. neonatal hypomagnesaemia
3. Excessive non-renal losses
   a. prolonged nasogastric suction
   b. laxative abuse
   c. intestinal/biliary fistulae
   d. chronic diarrhoea
   e. prolonged lactation (rare)
4. Excessive renal losses
   a. diuretic therapy
   b. diuretic phase of ATN
   c. chronic alcoholism
   d. primary hyperaldosteronism
   e. hypercalcaemia
   f. renal tubular acidosis
   g. diabetes
   h. hyperthyroidism
   i. aminoglycoside toxicity
   j. cis—platinum
   k. cyclosporin A
5. Miscellaneous
   a. idiopathic hypomagnesaemia
   b. acute pancreatitis
   c. acute porphyria with SIADH
   d. multiple transfusions of citrated blood.

Reduced intake of magnesium
This is probably the commonest cause of hypomagnesaemia in hospitalised patients where reduced dietary intake, e.g. postoperatively, is combined with the administration of large amounts of magnesium free fluids.

Reduced intestinal absorption
This is seen with all malabsorption syndromes and in patients who have had extensive small bowel resection. Neonatal hypomagnesaemia is due to selective failure of magnesium absorption. It presents with tetany, hypocalcaemia and seizures.

Excessive non-renal losses of magnesium
These occur principally from the gastrointestinal tract. Although gastric and biliary fluid contains very little magnesium, prolonged loss of these fluids can provoke hypomagnesaemia especially if intake is poor. Intestinal magnesium losses are greater, especially in chronic ulcerative colitis, Crohn's disease or chronic laxative abuse.

Excessive renal losses of magnesium
These occur in a large number of clinical situations. All diuretic states lead to considerable renal losses of magnesium. Alcohol has a direct effect on increasing urinary magnesium while the hypomagnesaemia seen during delirum tremens is aggravated by movement of magnesium into cells as a result of the accompanying respiratory alkalosis. Hypomagnesaemia in diabetics is seen typically during treatment of ketoacidosis, where insulin therapy increases urinary magnesium excretion. Severe hypomagnesaemia has recently been reported in renal transplant recipients receiving cyclosporin A and may contribute to the paraesthesiae that such patients frequently experience.

Miscellaneous
Miscellaneous causes of hypomagnesaemia include *acute intermittent porphyria* in which hypomagnesaemia is thought to be due to dilution from the accompanying SIADH.

Clinical features of hypomagnesaemia
Specific features of hypomagnesaemia are hard to define since it is frequently accompanied by hypocalcaemia and/or hypokalaemia. The main symptoms and signs are:

1. Neuromuscular
   a. muscle tremor/fibrillation
   b. carpopedal spasm
   c. tetany
   d. hyperreflexia
2. Neurological
   a. ataxia/vertigo
   b. depression/irritability
3. General—anorexia, nausea

4. Laboratory
   a. hypomagnesaemia, hypocalcaemia, hypokalaemia
   b. ECG—prolonged QT; broad, low T waves
   c. EMG—myopathic

These symptoms are accompanied and at times obscured by the symptoms and signs of the underlying cause. A high index of clinical suspicion is therefore required to enable the diagnosis to be made.

Therapy of hypomagnesaemia
Symptomatic hypomagnesaemia or magnesium depletion requires therapy. Magnesium replacement is given orally or intravenously, usually as magnesium sulphate. The amount required can be calculated simply. If hypomagnesaemia is severe (< 0.5 mmol/l) the magnesium deficit will be 0.5–1 mmol/kg. In replacing magnesium, twice this amount should be given as about half of any magnesium given will be lost in the urine even in severe magnesium depletion. The rate of I.V. administration should not exceed 50 mmol in 12 hours. Care should be exercised in replacing magnesium by the I.V. route in renal failure because of the risk of hypermagnesaemia. Frequent measurement of serum magnesium is required in such cases.

Appendix: Fluid, electrolyte and acid-base problems

Question 1

A middle-aged man was admitted to hospital with a 3 day history of watery diarrhoea. The following laboratory data were obtained.

	Day 1	Day 2
Na	130 mmol/l	137 mmol/l
K	2.5 mmol/l	4.2 mmol/l
Cl	115 mmol/l	114 mmol/l
HCO_3	5 mmol/l	13 mmol/l
urea	33.2 mmol/l	21 mmol/l
creatinine	390 umol/l	196 umol/l
pH	7.24	7.52
Pa_{CO2}	2.59 kPa	3.25 kPa
Pa_{O2}	15.3 kPa	14.3 kPa

1a. What is the acid-base abnormality on day 1?
1b. What is the aetiology of this acid-base abnormality?
1c. What is the acid-base abnormality on day 2?
1d. What is the aetiology of this acid-base abnormality?

Question 2

A 55 year-old male inhabitant of a home for the mentally
retarded was admitted after several days of 'feeling unwell'. He
had been tachypneic at rest and was drowsy. Physical
examination: T 39°C, P 108/min, BP 90/60, respirations 48/min.
Chest examination revealed signs of a left lower lobe pneumonia.
The following laboratory data were obtained at the time of his
admission:

Na	160 mmol/l	pH	7.13
K	8.4 mmol/l	Pa_{O_2}	7.03 kPa
Cl	133 mmol/l	Pa_{CO_2}	4.38 kPa
HCO_3	11 mmol/l		
Urea	62.6 mmol/l		
Creatinine	759 umol/l		
Glucose	5.3 mmol/l		

2a. What acid-base disorder(s) is (are) present?
2b. What is the aetiology of the hypernatraemia? Is total body
sodium likely to be high, normal or low?
2c. What is the aetiology of the hyperkalaemia?
2d. What immediate management is required?

Question 3

A 49 year-old woman was admitted following an overdose of an
unknown drug. She was stuporous and tachypneic. The following
laboratory data were obtained:

Na	140 mmol/l	pH	7.45
K	4.1 mmol/l	Pa_{CO_2}	1.8 kPa
Cl	109 mmol/l	Pa_{O_2}	15.3 kPa
HCO_3	9 mmol/l		
Urea	4.1 mmol/l		
Creatinine	130 umol/l		

3a. What is the acid-base disturbance?
3b. What is the likely aetiology?

Question 4

A 35 year-old man was admitted for elective inguinal herniorrhaphy. He was found to be mildly hypertensive (BP 160/100). Preoperative routine biochemistry revealed:

Serum			Urine		
Na	145 mmol/l		Na	45 mmol/l
Cl	95 mmol/l		K	40 mmol/l
K	2.8 mmol/l		Cl	50 mmol/l
HCO₃	33 mmol/l		pH	6.0
pH	7.5			
Pa_{CO2}	5.3 kPa			

4a. What acid-base disturbance is present?
4b. What is the aetiology of the hypokalaemia?
4c. What is the likely diagnosis?

Question 5

A 32 year-old man on treatment for hypertension was noted to have mild proteinuria and a urine sediment that contained occasional hyaline and granular casts and free fat. His renal function was normal and he had no oedema. Serum cholesterol was 7.2 mmol/l (normal 3.6–7.8 mmol/l) and triglycerides 6.16 mmol/l (0.28–1.69 mmol/l). After an unsuccessful attempt at controlling his hypertriglyceridaemia by diet he was placed on clofibrate 500 mg t.i.d. A month later he was admitted to hospital with complaints of feeling bloated, difficulty in concentrating and severe leg cramps. His wife reported that the day before admission he had seemed a little confused and that his urine output was diminished. The following laboratory data were obtained:

Serum		Urine	
Na	115 mmol/l	Na	80 mmol/l
K	4.0 mmol/l	Osmolality	486 mosm/kgH₂O
Cl	80 mmol/l		
HCO₃	22 mmol/l		
Urea	2.8 mmol/l		
creatinine	108 umol/l		
glucose	3.9 mmol/l		

5a. What is the pathophysiology of his hyponatraemia?
5b. How should the hyponatraemia be treated?

Question 6

An 8 year-old Asian boy, weight 24 kg, presents with proximal muscle weakness, bone pains and bilateral genu valgus. The following laboratory data were obtained:

serum		
	Ca	1.72 mmol/l
	P_{O_4}	0.61 mmol/l
	albumin	36 g/l
	AAT	22 U/l
	bilirubin	3.1 umol/l
	γ GT	16 U/l
	alkaline phosphatase	692U/l
	PTH	1864 pg/ml (normal up to 650 pg/ml)
24 hr urine	Ca	1.6 mmol/l
	P_{O_4}	28 mmol/l

6a. What is the most likely diagnosis?
6b. What is the aetiology of the hypophosphatemia and hypocalcaemia?

Question 7

A 56 year-old woman is being followed for moderate hypertension. She has no symptoms of note. The following laboratory data were obtained at a routine clinic visit:

serum				
	Na	140 mmol/l	Ca	2.94 mmol/l
	K	3.4 mmol/l	P_{O_4}	0.86 mmol/l
	Cl	113 mmol/l	albumin	40 g/l
	HCO_3	19 mmol/l	alkaline phosphatase	83 U/l
	urea	8.6 mmol/l	PTH	1486 pg/ml
	creatinine	156 umol/l		(normal up to 650 pg/ml)

7a. What diagnoses are likely?
7b What is the treatment of choice?

ANSWERS TO ACID-BASE/ELECTROLYTE PROBLEMS

1a. This patient has a normal anion-gap type metabolic acidosis (anion gap = $Na - (Cl + HCO_3)$ = 130 − 120 = 10 mmol/l). The Pa_{CO_2} has fallen by about 2.5 kPa which is appropriate for the fall in plasma bicarbonate.

1b. The systemic acidosis in this patient results from loss of bicarbonate in diarrhoea. He is volume contracted and has pre-renal azotaemia (urea = 33.2 mmol/l; creatinine = 390 umol/l; plasma urea/creatinine ratio = 85).

1c. On day 2 there is now a respiratory alkalosis (high pH, low Pa_{CO_2}). The fall in Pa_{CO_2} is appropriate for the observed reduction in plasma bicarbonate.

1d. The respiratory alkalosis is due to overrapid correction of the metabolic acidosis with bicarbonate. Persistent acidosis within the CSF (which takes several days to re-equilibrate) leads to hyperventilation and subsequent respiratory alkalosis.

2a. This patient has a mixed acid-base disorder. He has an increased anion-gap type of metabolic acidosis (anion gap = 16 mmol/l) related to his renal failure and/or lactic acidosis on the basis of fever, hypotension and hypoxaemia. In addition he has an acute respiratory acidosis since the observed Pa_{CO_2} (4.38 kPa) is inappropriately high for the Pa_{CO_2} expected (2.87–3.75 kPa) from the observed fall in plasma bicarbonate.

2b. The hypernatraemia results from severe volume depletion due to a combination of fever, hyperventilation and inadequate fluid intake. Plasma volume, in this situation, is maintained at the expense of serum osmolality. His calculated serum osmolality is 303 mosm/kg H_2O. Total body sodium is likely to be low.

2c. The hyperkalaemia is multifactorial in origin with renal failure, systemic acidosis and hypoxic tissue damage all contributing.

2d. The main threats to this patient's life are from acidosis, hyperkalaemia, severe volume depletion and renal failure. Urgent therapy for the hyperkalaemia should be undertaken while the other problems are being assessed and treated. The hyperkalaemia should be treated with intravenous Ca gluconate 10–20 ml 10%, sodium bicarbonate 50–100 mmol (50–100 ml 8.4%) and oral or rectal Ca Resonium 15–30 g. In addition an infusion of glucose 25 g (50 ml 50%) and soluble insulin 10 U will promote redistribution of potassium into cells.

The hypovalaemia requires rehydration with 0.9% or 0.45% NaCl. The volume given should be assessed by physical examination, calculation of the volume deficit and direct measurement of central venous or pulmonary wedge pressures. Correction of the hypernatraemia should proceed slowly at no more than 2 mosm/kg H_2O hourly.

The man has severe azotaemia. It is likely that he has established acute renal failure which could readily be confirmed by checking a 'spot' urine Na and/or osmolality. If so he will require urgent haemodialysis. This is in any case indicated for the acidosis and severe hyperkalaemia. He should be haemodialysed against a high dialysate sodium (145 mmol/l) to prevent disequilibrium.

3a. This patient has a mixed acid-base disturbance. She has an increased anion-gap type metabolic acidosis (anion gap = 22 mmol/l). In addition she has a respiratory alkalosis since her Pa_{CO_2} at 1.9 kPa is lower than the Pa_{CO_2} expected (2.5–3.47 kPa) for the 15 mmol/l fall in her plasma bicarbonate. For this reason the final blood pH is alkalaemic.

3b. In the absence of renal failure the clinical history is most consistent with salicylate intoxication.

4a. This patient has a hypokalaemic metabolic alkalosis. The normal Pa_{CO_2} is consistent with this diagnosis.

4b. From the laboratory data given the hypokalaemia is the result of renal potassium loss. Since the patient is not on diuretics this suggests a mineralocorticoid excess.

4c. In this hypertensive young man Conn's syndrome is the most likely diagnosis. Cushing's syndrome, liquorice ingestion and carbonoxolone therapy should be excluded by history or appropriate laboratory tests.

5a. The likeliest explanation for this man's hyponatraemia is water intoxication resulting from SIADH. Pseudohyponatraemia due to his hyperlipidaemia is very unlikely since the magnitude of fall in serum sodium is too great. A rise in serum triglycerides of 2.5 mmol/l will normally cause a 1 mmol/l fall in serum sodium. Similarly hyperglycaemia can be ruled out as a cause of hyponatraemia. He is oedema free and there is no history to suggest volume depletion.

5b. The likely cause of his SIADH is the clofibrate. This should be stopped. Water restriction, would be expected to restore his serum sodium to normal in a few days. Since he is symptomatic it would also be correct to treat him with frusemide and hypertonic saline. After initiation of a diuresis his urinary sodium losses should be replaced as hypertonic saline resulting in net water loss. This will correct serum sodium within 12–24 hours.

6a. The most likely diagnosis given the ethnic background of the child and the clinical and laboratory data is nutritional vitamin D deficient rickets.

6b. The hypophosphataemia is due to phosphaturia caused by the secondary hyperparathyroidism that accompanies vitamin D deficiency. The hypocalcaemia is largely due to reduced intestinal calcium absorption. The very low urinary calcium supports this.

7a. The most likely diagnosis is primary hyperparathyroidism. This is supported by the hypercalcaemia, low normal phosphate, mild non-anion gap type metabolic acidosis and elevated PTH. Malignancy with ectopic PTH production is a possibility though unlikely in the absence of any other symptoms. Details of drug therapy are not given but the patient is hypertensive and could be on a thiazide diuretic. This may have caused her hypercalcaemia but does not exclude primary hyperparathyroidism.

7b. No therapy is needed at this time. However, her serum creatinine is mildly elevated suggesting possible nephrocalcinosis. If further investigation confirms this she should have a parathyroidectomy. If she is on a thiazide diuretic it should be stopped if possible.

Bibliography

Below is given a list of some of the comprehensive texts used in preparation of the manuscript to which the interested reader is directed. There follows also a list of selected Journal articles which cover most of the areas dealt with in the text and which have their emphasis on practical clinical considerations rather than basic physiology.

Textbooks
Valtin H 1983 Renal function. Mechanisms preserving fluid and solute balance in health (2nd Edn). Little Brown and Company, Boston

Schrier R W (Ed) 1980 Renal and electrolyte disorders (2nd Edn). Little Brown and Company, Boston

Schwarz A B, Lyons H (Eds) 1977 Acid-base and electrolyte balance. Grune and Stratton, New York

Brenner B M, Stein J H (Eds) 1978 Contemporary issues in nephrology 1. Sodium and water homeostasis. Churchill Livingstone, New York

Brenner B M, Stein J H (Eds) 1978 Contemporary issues in nephrology 2. Acid-base and potassium homeostasis. Churchill Livingstone, New York

Brenner B M, Stein J H (Eds) 1983 Contemporary issues in nephrology 11. Divalent ion homeostasis. Churchill Livingstone, New York

Suki W N, Massry S G (Eds) 1984 Therapy of renal diseases and related disorders. Martinus Nijhoff, Boston

Arieff A I, Defronzo R A (Eds) 1985 Fluid, electrolytes and acid-base disorders. Vols 1 and 2. Churchill Livingstone, New York

Journal articles
Narins R G et al 1982 Diagnostic strategies in disorders of fluid, electrolyte and acid-base homeostasis. American Journal of Medicine 72: 496–520

Bear R A, Neil G A 1984 A clinical approach to common electrolyte problems. 2. Potassium inbalances. Canadian Medical Association Journal 129: 28–31

Kurtzman N A 1983 Acquired distal renal tubular acidosis. Kidney International 24: 807–819

Harrington J T 1984 Metabolic alkalosis. Kidney International 25: 88–97

Gabow P A 1985 Disorders associated with an altered anion gap. Kidney International 27: 472–483

Berkelhammer C, Bear R A 1984 A clinical approach to common electrolyte problems. 3. Hypophosphatemia. Canadian Medical Association Journal 130:17–23

Dirks J H 1983 The kidney and magnesiuim regulation. Kidney
　　International 23: 771–777
Berkelhammer C, Bear R A 1985 A clinical approach to common
　　electrolyte problems. 4. Hypomagnesemia. Canadian Medical
　　Association Journal 132: 360–368.

Index